Healthy Recipes Top 46 Poultry Recipes

Learn How to Mix Different Ingredients to Create Tasty Meals and Build A Complete Meal Plan For Your Diet

Jane Sommers

Table of Contents

Introduction

1. Sun-Dried Tomato Chicken Pasta Salad

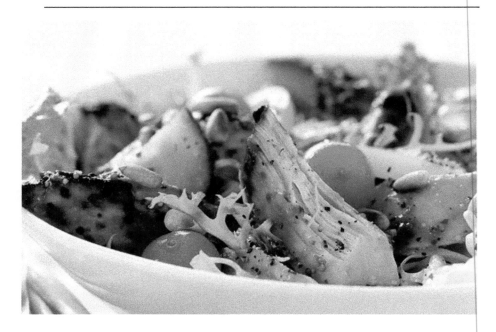

Prep Time: 15 Minutes

Cook Time: 8 Minutes

Total Time: 23 Minutes

Servings: 10

Ingredients

- 1 pound small dried pasta (any variety)
- 2 cups chopped leftover cooked chicken or rotisserie chicken
- 1 cup fresh baby spinach, packed
- 7 ounces sun-dried tomatoes in oil, drained
- 5 ounces pitted green olives, halved
- 1/3 cup chopped red onion
- 3/4 cup light mayonnaise

- 1/4 cup red wine vinegar
- 1 tablespoon dried Italian seasoning
- 1 clove garlic, peeled
- 1/4 teaspoon crushed red pepper

Instructions

- Place a large pot of salted water on the stovetop and bring to a boil. Cook the pasta according to package instructions. Drain the pasta in a colander and rinse with cold water to cool. Allow the paste to drain while you prep the remaining ingredients.
- Chop the sun-dried tomatoes into bite-sized pieces. Place the mayonnaise, red wine vinegar, Italian seasoning, garlic, crushed red pepper, and 1/4 cup chopped sun-dried tomatoes in the blender jar. Cover and puree.
- Place the cooled pasta, chopped chicken, spinach, remaining chopped sun-dried tomatoes, olives, and onions in a large salad bowl. Add the creamy dressing and toss to coat. Cover the bowl with plastic wrap and refrigerate until ready to serve.

Nutrition

Calories: 285kcal, Carbohydrates: 48g, Protein: 9g, Fat: 7g, Saturated Fat: 1g, Cholesterol: 2mg, Sodium: 401mg, Potassium: 823mg, Fiber: 4g, Sugar: 9g, Vitamin C: 9.1mg, Calcium: 52mg, Iron: 2.8mg

2. Instant Pot Sweet Soy Chicken Thighs

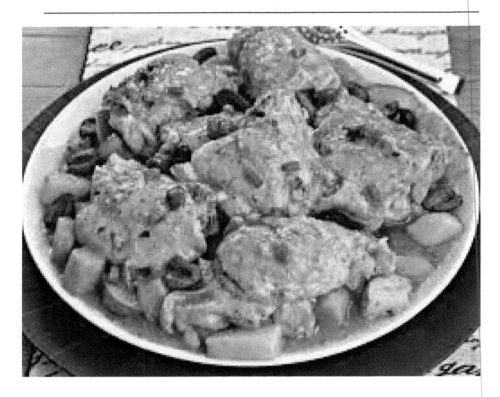

Prep Time: 5 Minutes

Cook Time: 35 Minutes

Total Time: 45 Minutes

Servings: 6

Ingredients

- 4 pounds bone-in chicken thighs (10-12 thighs)
- 1 cup low-sodium soy sauce (I bought gluten-free)
- 3/4 cup brown sugar, packed
- 1/4 cup ketchup

8

- 4 cloves garlic, minced
- 2 tablespoons fresh grated ginger
- 1 tablespoon sesame oil
- 1 tablespoon cornstarch or arrowroot
- Garnishes: sesame seeds and chopped scallions

Instructions

- Turn the Instant Pot on the Sauté setting and add the sesame oil. Add several of the chicken thighs, skin-side-down. Brown the skin for 2-3 minutes, until golden brown. Then remove the chicken thighs and repeat with the remaining thighs until all have been browned on the skin side. Place all the chicken thighs back in the Instant Pot, skin-side-up. This first step is optional. Then the skin will not stay crisp once pressure-cooked, but the browning process gives the skin a much richer color once finished. If skipping the browning, pile the raw thighs in the Instant Pot and move onto step 2.
- Pour the soy sauce, brown sugar, ketchup, garlic, and ginger into a bowl. Whisk well, then pour the glaze over the top of the chicken.
- Lock the lid into place. Set the Instant Pot on Pressure Cook High for 20 minutes. Then turn the Instant Pot Off and perform a Quick Release. Once the pressure valve button drops, it's safe to open the lid.
- Scoop 1/4 cup of the glaze out of the pot. Whisk 1 tablespoon cornstarch into the glaze. Then turn the Instant Pot back on Sauté and stir the cornstarch slurry back into the pot. Let it simmer for 2-4 minutes to thicken the glaze. Turn off the pot. Sprinkle with sesame seeds and chopped scallions before servings.

Nutrition

Calories: 831kcal, Carbohydrates: 36g, Protein: 51g, Fat: 52g, Saturated Fat: 13g, Cholesterol: 296mg, Sodium: 1748mg, Potassium: 782mg, Fiber: 0g, Sugar: 29g, Vitamin C: 1.1mg, Calcium: 58mg, Iron: 3.2mg

3. Pesto Chicken Baked Tortellini

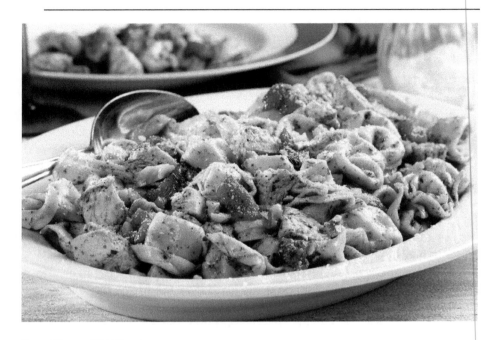

Prep Time: 10 Minutes

Cook Time: 40 Minutes

Total Time: 50 Minutes

Servings: 10

Ingredients

- 40 ounces cheese tortellini, refrigerated or frozen and thawed
- 1 pound boneless, skinless chicken breasts, chopped into 1 inch cubes
- 1 tablespoon butter
- 1 red bell pepper, seeded and chopped
- 1/2 red onion, peeled and chopped
- 6 ounces basil pesto or homemade pesto
- 2 cups fresh baby spinach
- 2 cups chicken broth

- 1 cup heavy cream
- 2 cups shredded fontina cheese
- 1/2 cup shaved Parmesan cheese
- Salt and pepper

Instructions

- Preheat the oven to 400 degrees F. Place the butter in a medium-sized skillet and set it on the stovetop over medium heat. Add the onions and sauté for 2 minutes. Then stir in the chopped red pepper and sauté for another 2 minutes. Turn off the heat.
- Pour the tortellini into a large 3-quart (9x13-inch) baking dish. Place the chopped chicken, fresh spinach, and sautéed onions and peppers in the dish. Toss to mix evenly and spread out in the pan.
- Mix the pesto, chicken broth, heavy cream, 1 teaspoon salt, and 1/2 teaspoon ground black pepper in a bowl or measuring pitcher. Whisk well, then pour the mixture over the tortellini.
- Cover the pan with foil and bake for 20 minutes. Then gently stir the pasta to make sure the tortellini on top is covered in sauce. Sprinkle the top with both kinds of cheese and bake, uncovered, for another 15-20 minutes. Serve warm.

Nutrition

Calories: 694kcal, Carbohydrates: 53g, Protein: 37g, Fat: 36g, Saturated Fat: 16g, Cholesterol: 143mg, Sodium: 1191mg, Potassium: 311mg, Fiber: 5g, Sugar: 4g, Vitamin C: 21.3mg, Calcium: 420mg, Iron: 3.6mg

4. Grilled Tex Mex Stuffed Avocado Recipe

Prep Time: 5 Minutes

Cook Time: 5 Minutes

Total Time: 10 Minutes

Servings: 8 Halves

Ingredients

- 4 ripe avocados
- 16 ounces Old El Paso Refried Beans
- 10 ounces Old El Paso Red Enchilada Sauce
- 1 cup shredded cooked chicken (use leftovers or a rotisserie chicken)
- 1 cup shredded Mexican blend cheese (could be reduced fat)
- 1/4 cup crumbled queso fresco
- 1/4 cup chopped green onions

Instructions

- Preheat the grill to high heat. Slice the avocados in half, lengthwise, and remove the pits. Lay the avocados on the grill(cut side down) and grill for 2 minutes.
- Take the avocados off the grill and turn them over. Dollop 1-2 tablespoons of refried beans in the center of each avocado. Then top with shredded chicken, a generous spoonful of enchilada sauce, and shredded cheese.
- Grill the avocados with the fillings up, for another 2-3 minutes, until the fillings are warm and the cheese has melted.
- Sprinkle with crumbled queso fresco and chopped green onions. Serve warm.

Nutrition

Calories: 305kcal, Carbohydrates: 18g, Protein: 11g, Fat: 21g, Saturated Fat: 5g, Cholesterol: 26mg, Sodium: 776mg, Potassium:

539mg, Fiber: 9g, Sugar: 4g, Vitamin C: 11.6mg, Calcium: 148mg, Iron: 1.5mg

257. Peruvian Baked Chicken And Vegetable Roll-Ups

Prep Time: 15 Minutes

Cook Time: 30 Minutes

Total Time: 45 Minutes

Servings: 8 Rolls

Ingredients

- 2 pounds chicken breast cutlets (8 cutlets)
- 1 teaspoon ground cumin
- 1 teaspoon smoked paprika
- 1 teaspoon dried oregano
- 1/4 teaspoon garlic powder
- 2 plantains
- 2 bell peppers, any color
- 1 bunch scallions
- 2 tablespoons olive oil
- Salt and pepper
- Aji Verde Sauce

Instructions

- Preheat the oven to 425 degrees F. Line a large rimmed baking sheet with parchment paper.
- Trim the ends off the plantains and score a shallow line from end to end, to open the peel. Gently pull off the peel in sections. Then cut the plantains in half, and cut each half into quarters lengthwise, creating 8 french fry-shaped strips per plantain.
- Cut the bell peppers in half. Remove the seeds, then cut the peppers into strips, 1/2-inch inch wide. Trim the root ends off the scallions, then cut them in half, so that all the produce is about the same length.

- Place the plantains and peppers on the baking sheet. Sprinkle with salt and roast in the oven for 15 minutes.
- Meanwhile, mix the cumin, paprika, oregano, garlic powder, 1 teaspoon salt, and 1/4 teaspoon ground black pepper in a small bowl. Sprinkle the spice mix over the chicken cutlets, coating both sides.
- After the plantains and peppers are partially cooked, lay 2-4 pieces of each across each chicken cutlet. (Larger cutlets will hold more.) Fold the ends of the chicken over the produce and fasten tightly with a toothpick. Lay the finished rolls on the baking sheet.
- Bake for 15-20 minutes until the thickest part of the chicken is cooked through. Serve warm, topped with fresh zesty Aji Verde sauce.

Nutrition

Calories: 195kcal, Carbohydrates: 8g, Protein: 24g, Fat: 6g, Saturated Fat: 1g, Cholesterol: 72mg, Sodium: 133mg, Potassium: 595mg, Fiber: 1g, Sugar: 4g, Vitamin A: 315iu, Vitamin C: 28.4mg, Calcium: 19mg, Iron: 1mg

5. Chicken Minestrone Soup

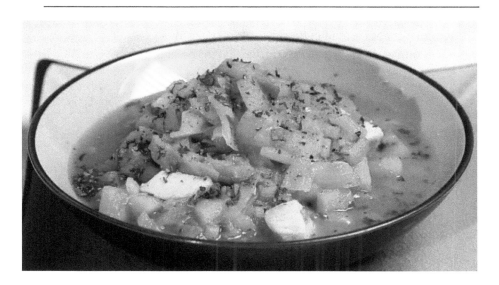

Prep Time: 10 Minutes

Cook Time: 35 Minutes

Total Time: 45 Minutes

Servings: 8

Ingredients

- 1 1/4 pounds boneless, skinless chicken breast
- 2 tablespoons olive oil
- 1 large onion, peeled and chopped
- 6 cloves garlic, minced
- 8 ounces button mushrooms, sliced
- 2 carrots, sliced
- 6 cups chicken broth
- 6 cups water
- 2 cans fire-roasted diced tomatoes (15-ounce cans)
- 1/2 cup red wine
- 2 tablespoons dried Italian seasoning

- 1 small zucchini, quartered and sliced
- 1 small summer squash, quartered and sliced
- 15 ounces kidney beans, drained (1 can)
- 15 ounces cannellini beans, drained (1 can)
- 8 ounce dried macaroni noodles (could be gluten-free)
- 1 cup frozen cut green beans
- 1/2 cup chopped roasted red peppers
- Salt and pepper

Instructions

- Set a large 6-8 quart soup pot over medium heat. Add the olive oil, onions, garlic, mushrooms, and carrots. Sauté for 5-8 minutes to soften the vegetables, stirring regularly.
- Place the whole chicken breasts down in the sautéed veggies at the bottom of the pot. Add in the chicken broth, water, canned tomatoes, red wine, Italian seasoning, 1 teaspoon salt, and 1/4 teaspoon ground black pepper. Bring to a boil and simmer for 15-20 minutes, until the chicken breasts are cooked through.
- Remove the chicken breasts with tongs and set them on a cutting board. Add the zucchini, summer squash, canned beans, macaroni, green beans, and roasted red peppers to the pot. Stir well. Bring to a simmer and cook for another 5-8 minutes, until the pasta is cooked through.
- Meanwhile, chop the chicken into bite-size pieces. Stir the chicken back into the soup. Taste, then salt and pepper as needed.

Nutrition

Calories: 338kcal, Carbohydrates: 43g, Protein: 25g, Fat: 6g, Saturatedfat: 1g, Cholesterol: 45mg, Sodium: 1147mg, Potassium: 839mg, Fiber: 6g, Sugar: 6g, Vitamin A: 3240iu, Vitamin C: 32.6mg, Calcium: 137mg, Iron: 3.9mg

6. Honey Orange Roasted Chicken Recipe

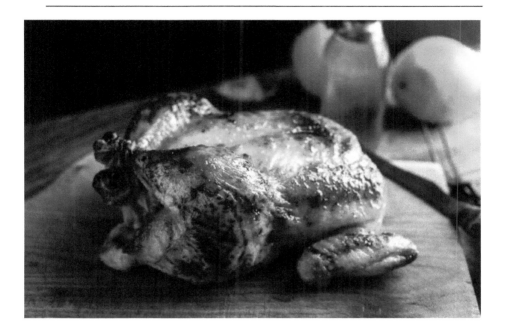

Prep Time: 10 Minutes

Cook Time: 2 Hours

Total Time: 2 Hours 10 Minutes

Servings: 6

Ingredients

For The Honey Orange Roast Chicken:

- 7-8 pound chicken, whole
- 1/2 cup unsalted butter, softened
- 1/4 cup honey

- 1 small orange, such as a clementine
- Salt and pepper
- For the Honey Orange Gravy:
- Pan juices from the chicken
- 3 tablespoons flour
- 2 cups chicken stock
- Salt and pepper

For The Grilled Spring Veggies:

- 12 ounces thin french green beans (haricot vert) trimmed
- 12 ounces thin baby asparagus, trimmed
- Salt and pepper

Instructions

- Preheat the oven to 450 degrees F. Remove the neck and gizzards from inside the chicken. Place the chicken in a small dry skillet and pat the skin dry with paper towels. Slide a regular tablespoon, curved side down, underneath the skin of the chicken. Run the spoon along the breast to loosen the skin on both sides, and down over the drumsticks. Then mix the butter, honey, and the zest of one orange with 3/4 teaspoon salt and 1/4 teaspoon black pepper. Mash the ingredients in a small bowl until well combined. Use the spoon to deposit the butter mixture underneath the skin of the chicken. Place as much of the butter as possible over the breast meat and drumsticks. Then press the skin to smooth. Rub any remaining butter over the outside of the skin and sprinkle with salt and pepper. Slice the orange and place it inside the chicken.
- Roast the chicken for 45 minutes to crisp up the skin, then lower the heat to 350 degrees F. If the skin is brown, cover the chicken loosely with foil and continue roasting for another 75 - 90 minutes. (My chicken was exactly 8 pounds and it was finished in 2 hours total.) To test the chicken for doneness, stick a knife down between the drumstick and the breast. If the juices run out clear, the chicken is ready.
- Remove the chicken from the oven and carefully lift it out of the juices. Place it on a platter and cover with foil to keep it warm.
- While the chicken is roasting, place a large grill pan over two burners and turn them both on medium heat. Lay the asparagus and green

beans on the grill pan and sear until the color has intensified and grill marks have formed. Flip once and salt and pepper. Cook the veggies until just cooked through, so they are bright green and firm. Approximately 6-10 minutes.

- Place the sauté pan with the chicken juices over another burner. Heat the burner to medium heat and whisk in the flour. Add the chicken stock, then salt and pepper to taste. (You may need as much as 3/4 teaspoon salt, depending on how salty the juices and stock are. Start with a little salt and add more.) Bring the gravy to a boil and whisk. Continue simmering and stirring until the gravy is thick enough to coat a spoon.
- To Serve: Cut the chicken into pieces and distribute it onto plates. Spoon the grilled veggies next to the chicken and drizzle honey orange gravy over both the chicken and veggies.

Nutrition

Calories: 806kcal, Carbohydrates: 26g, Protein: 52g, Fat: 54g, Saturated Fat: 20g, Cholesterol: 233mg, Sodium: 299mg, Potassium: 845mg, Fiber: 3g, Sugar: 17g, Vitamin A: 1695iu, Vitamin C: 25.9mg, Calcium: 78mg, Iron: 4.5mg

7. Pollo Rojo (Red Pepper Chicken)

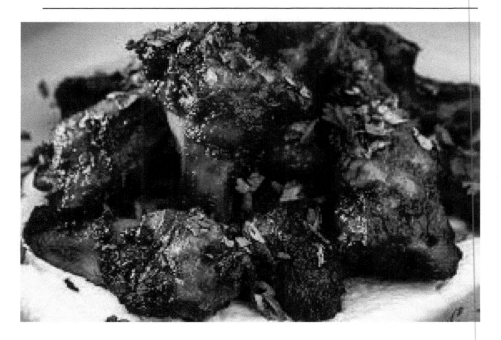

Prep Time: 25 Minutes

Cook Time: 10 Minutes

Total Time: 35 Minutes

Servings: 4

Ingredients

For The Red Pepper Mole:

- 14-15 dried New Mexico chiles, Anaheims or California
- 2 cloves garlic
- 1 cup chicken stock (any stock would work)
- 1 tablespoon ground cumin
- 2 tablespoons honey
- 3 tablespoons rice vinegar
- 1/2 teaspoon salt

- For the Red Pepper Chicken:
- 2 pounds chicken cutlets (thinly sliced breast meat)
- 1 tablespoon oil
- 1 tablespoon butter
- Salt and pepper

Instructions

- Prepare a bowl of boiling water. Place the chiles in the water and allow them to soak for 10-15 minutes, until soft to the touch.
- Remove the stems, seeds, and membranes, rinsing each pepper in the bowl. Then place in a food processor.
- Add the garlic cloves and half the chicken stock. Puree until smooth. Then add the cumin, honey, vinegar, salt, and remaining stock. Puree again until smooth. Taste and salt again if needed. The sauce should have a very intense flavor, but not be overly spicy if the seeds and membranes are properly removed.
- Heat a large to medium-high heat. Pat the chicken cutlets dry and salt the pepper on both sides.
- Add the oil and butter to the skillet. Once melted, place half the cutlets in the pan. Saute for 2-3 minutes per side. Repeat with the remaining cutlets.
- To Serve: Warm the red pepper sauce and pour over the chicken. Garnish with cilantro leaves or queso fresco.

Nutrition

Calories: 441kcal, Carbohydrates: 25g, Protein: 53g, Fat: 13g, Saturated Fat: 3g, Cholesterol: 154mg, Sodium: 682mg, Potassium: 1436mg, Fiber: 2g, Sugar: 17g, Vitamin C: 229.5mg, Calcium: 50mg, Iron: 3.6mg

8. Healthy Chicken Cacciatore Soup

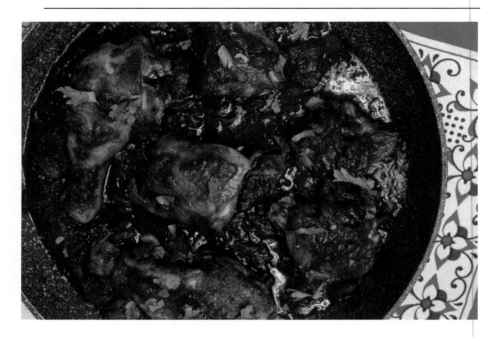

Prep Time: 15 Minutes

Cook Time: 30 Minutes

Total Time: 45 Minutes

Servings: 10

Ingredients

- 2 boneless, skinless chicken breasts, cubed
- 1 tablespoon olive oil
- 1 tablespoon butter
- 4-6 cloves garlic, minced
- 1 large onion, chopped
- 1 cup celery, chopped
- 1 cup carrots, chopped
- 1 medium zucchini, chopped

22

- 8 ounces mushrooms (cremini or button), sliced
- 2 cans diced tomatoes, (2 cans) with garlic and herbs for added flavor
- 28 ounces tomato sauce
- 6 cups chicken stock
- 1 cup wine, white or red
- 1/8-1/4 teaspoon crushed red pepper flakes
- 1 tablespoon Italian seasonings
- 1 bunch fresh basil leaves
- 2 cups small dried pasta
- 1 cup shredded Parmesan cheese
- Salt and pepper

Instructions

- In a large stock, pot browns the chicken in oil and butter over medium heat.
- Add the garlic, onions, celery, and carrots. Sauté for 3-5 minutes, then and 1 cup of the stock simmering for 3 minutes.
- Add everything except the fresh basil, Parmesan cheese, and pasta. Stir in 1 teaspoon salt and 1/2 teaspoon ground black pepper. Simmer for 10 minutes.
- Add the pasta and half of the fresh basil. Simmer for 8-10 more minutes until the pasta is al dente. At this point add 1-2 cups of water if needed. Stir in Parmesan cheese.
- Garnish with a sprinkle of Parmesan cheese and more fresh basil.

Nutrition

Calories: 259kcal, Carbohydrates: 27g, Protein: 16g, Fat: 8g, Saturatedfat: 3g, Cholesterol: 28mg, Sodium: 849mg, Potassium: 929mg, Fiber: 3g, Sugar: 10g, Vitamin A: 2840iu, Vitamin C: 20.1mg, Calcium: 190mg, Iron: 2.8mg

9. Skillet Chicken Puttanesca

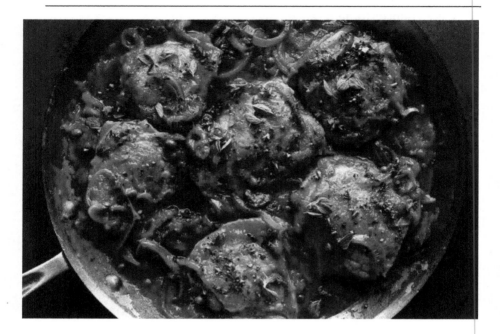

Prep Time: 5 Minutes

Cook Time: 18 Minutes

Total Time: 23 Minutes

Servings: 4

Ingredients

- 4 boneless skinless chicken breasts
- 2 tablespoons olive oil
- 3 cloves garlic, minced
- 8 anchovy fillets, minced (from a small can)
- 28 ounces crushed tomatoes
- 1/4 cup chopped parsley
- 1 1/2 teaspoon dried oregano
- 1/2 teaspoon crushed red pepper

- 6 ounces pitted kalamata olives, drained
- 3 ounces pitted green olives, drained
- 3 ounces capers, drained
- Salt and pepper

Instructions

- Set a large sauté pan over medium-high heat. Season the chicken on both sides with salt and pepper. Add the oil to the pan and cook the chicken breasts for 4-5 minutes per side. Remove the chicken from the skillet and set it aside.
- Next, add the garlic and anchovies to the skillet. Sauté for 2 minutes, then pour in the tomatoes, parsley, oregano, and crushed red pepper. Stir well, and add in the olives and capers. Simmer 8-10 minutes.
- Place the chicken back into the sauce. Simmer the chicken for 3-4 minutes to heat through. Serve warm as a low carb meal, or serve with pasta.

Nutrition

Calories: 369kcal, Carbohydrates: 19g, Protein: 30g, Fat: 20g, Saturated Fat: 3g, Cholesterol: 77mg, Sodium: 1989mg, Potassium: 1096mg, Fiber: 7g, Sugar: 9g, Vitamin A: 1145iu, Vitamin C: 26.2mg, Calcium: 148mg, Iron: 4.4mg

10. Skinny Creamy Chimichurri Chicken Skillet

Prep Time: 5 Minutes

Cook Time: 13 Minutes

Total Time: 18 Minutes

Servings: 4

Ingredients

- 4 boneless skinless chicken breasts
- 1 tablespoon olive oil
- 1 bunch parsley, stems removed
- 1/2 onion, cut into wedges
- 2 cloves garlic
- 3 ounces fat-free cream cheese
- 3 tablespoons red wine vinegar
- 1 tablespoon dried oregano
- 1 1/2 teaspoons ground cumin
- 1/4 teaspoon crushed red pepper
- 1 cup water
- Salt and pepper

Instructions

- Place a large deep skillet over medium heat and add the oil. Season the chicken breasts with salt and pepper. Once the skillet is hot add the chicken breasts and cook 4 minutes per side.
- Meanwhile, peel the onion and garlic cloves. Place the parsley, onion, garlic, vinegar, oregano, cumin, crushed red pepper, and 1/2 teaspoon salt in the food processor. Pulse until the mixture is well chopped. Then add in the cream cheese and water. Turn on and puree until very smooth.
- Once the chicken has seared for 4 minutes per side, pour the sauce over the chicken. Simmer for 3-5 minutes to let the chicken finish

cooking and the sauce thicken. Taste, then salt and pepper as needed.

Nutrition

Calories: 253kcal, Carbohydrates: 4g, Protein: 26g, Fat: 14g, Saturated Fat: 5g, Cholesterol: 95mg, Sodium: 215mg, Potassium: 575mg, Fiber: 1g, Sugar: 1g, Vitamin C: 21.8mg, Calcium: 79mg, Iron: 2.4mg

11.   Skinny Creamy Chicken Broccoli Soup

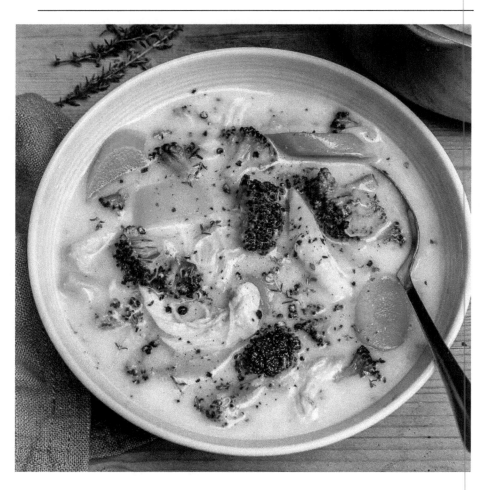

Prep Time: 10 Minutes

Cook Time: 25 Minutes

Total Time: 35 Minutes

Servings: 6

Ingredients

- ❖ 1 large onion, chopped
- 3 cloves garlic, minced
- 1 tablespoon butter
- 1 pound boneless skinless chicken breast
- 8 cups low-sodium chicken broth
- 3 tablespoons dry sherry
- 2 tablespoons Dijon mustard
- 1 teaspoon cornstarch
- 1/2 teaspoons smoked paprika
- 1/4 teaspoon crushed red pepper
- 4 ounces fat-free cream cheese, cut into cubes
- 3 cups small fresh broccoli florets
- Salt and pepper
- Possible Garnishes: Low fat shredded cheese, chopped scallions, fresh parsley

Instructions

- Place the butter in a 4-quart soup pot and set over medium heat. Once the butter has melted, add the onions and garlic. Sauté for 3-4 minutes, stirring to make sure the garlic doesn't burn.
- Place the whole chicken breasts at the bottom of the pot. Add the broth, sherry, Dijon mustard, corn starch, smoked paprika, crushed red pepper, 1 teaspoon salt, and 1/2 teaspoon ground black pepper.
- Bring the broth to a boil. Lower the heat, cover, and simmer for 15-20 minutes to cook the chicken.
- Remove the chicken breast with tongs. Then add in the cream cheese. Whisk to melt the cream cheese into the broth. Then use two forks to shred the chicken.
- Add the broccoli florets and the shredded chicken to the soup. Stir well and turn off the heat. The small broccoli florets will cook quickly in the hot broth.
- Taste, then salt and pepper as needed. Serve warm.

Nutrition

Calories: 254kcal, Carbohydrates: 10g, Protein: 25g, Fat: 12g, Saturated Fat: 5g, Cholesterol: 74mg, Sodium: 334mg, Potassium:

759mg, Fiber: 1g, Sugar: 2g, Vitamin C: 43.3mg, Calcium: 66mg, Iron: 1.5mg

12. Low Carb Green Curry Chicken Noodle Soup

Prep Time: 10 Minutes

Cook Time: 25 Minutes

Total Time: 35 Minutes

Servings: 8

Ingredients

- 1 teaspoon coconut oil
- 1 onion, peeled and chopped
- 3 cloves garlic, minced
- 1 tablespoon fresh grated ginger
- 1 red bell pepper, seeded and chopped
- 3 carrots, sliced
- 1 1/4 pounds whole boneless skinless chicken breast
- 13.5 ounces thick unsweetened coconut milk (1 can)
- 3-6 tablespoons green curry paste
- 9 cups chicken broth
- 3 tablespoons fish sauce
- 14 ounces konnyaku noodles
- 2 cups small broccoli florets
- 1/2 cup fresh Thai basil leaves
- Salt and pepper

Instructions

- Place the oil in a large 6-8 quart saucepot over medium heat. Once the oil is hot, sauté the onions, minced garlic, and ginger for 3 minutes to soften. Stir in the chopped bell pepper and carrots.
- Add the chicken breasts, coconut milk, 3 tablespoons green curry paste, chicken broth, and fish sauce to the pot. Raise the heat to high and bring to a boil. Once boiling, reduce the heat back to medium, then simmer for 15 minutes.

- Meanwhile, drain and rinse the konnyaku noodles.
- Using tongs, remove the chicken breasts from the pot. Use a fork and tongs to shred the chicken. Then place it back in the pot. Stir in the konnyaku noodles and the broccoli florets. Taste, then add 1-3 more tablespoons green curry paste if desired. Taste again, then salt and pepper as needed.
- Garnish with fresh basil leaves and serve warm.

Nutrition

Calories: 231kcal, Carbohydrates: 9g, Protein: 18g, Fat: 13g, Saturated Fat: 10g, Cholesterol: 45mg, Sodium: 1610mg, Potassium: 803mg, Fiber: 1g, Sugar: 3g, Vitamin C: 62.6mg, Calcium: 65mg, Iron: 3mg

13.   The Best Thai Panang Chicken Curry

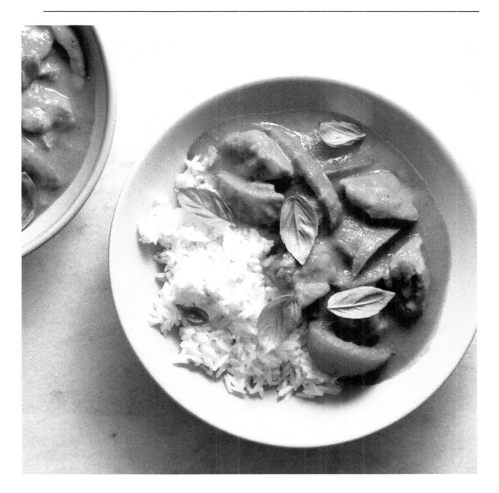

Prep Time: 10 Minutes

Cook Time: 22 Minutes

Total Time: 32 Minutes

Servings: 6

Ingredients

- 1 1/2 pounds boneless skinless chicken thighs chopped
- 1 small onion, peeled and chopped
- 1 red bell pepper, seeded and chopped
- 1 orange bell pepper, seeded and chopped
- 2 cloves garlic, minced
- 1 tablespoon coconut oil
- 4 ounces Panang red curry paste (1 can)
- 1 tablespoon peanut butter
- 12 kaffir lime leaves, crushed
- 13.5 ounces thick coconut milk, unsweetened (1 can)
- 3 tablespoons fish sauce
- 1/4 cup Thai basil leaves or sweet basil

Instructions

- Cut the chicken into bite-size pieces. Chop the onions and peppers into roughly 1-inch pieces. Mince the garlic. Then crush the kaffir lime leaves to help release their oils.
- Place a 14-inch skillet (or wok) over medium-high heat. Add the coconut oil. Once the oil melts, add the onions. Sauté for 1 minute, then add the peppers and garlic. Sauté another 2-3 minutes.
- Move the veggies to the sides of the skillet and add the Panang red curry paste and peanut butter to the center of the pan. Sauté the curry for 2-3 minutes to intensify the flavor, moving around the pan. Then add the kaffir lime leaves, coconut milk, and fish sauce. Stir to blend.
- Stir in the chopped chicken and bring to a boil. Lower the heat and simmer for 10-15 minutes, until the chicken is cooked through and the sauce thickens. Stir occasionally. Remove from heat and stir in the basil leaves. Serve with rice, quinoa, or noodles.

Nutrition

Calories: 340kcal, Carbohydrates: 8g, Protein: 24g, Fat: 23g, Saturated Fat: 16g, Cholesterol: 107mg, Sodium: 163mg, Potassium: 545mg, Fiber: 2g, Sugar: 4g, Vitamin C: 54.7mg, Calcium: 56mg, Iron: 3.8mg

14.   Spicy Thai Chicken Soup

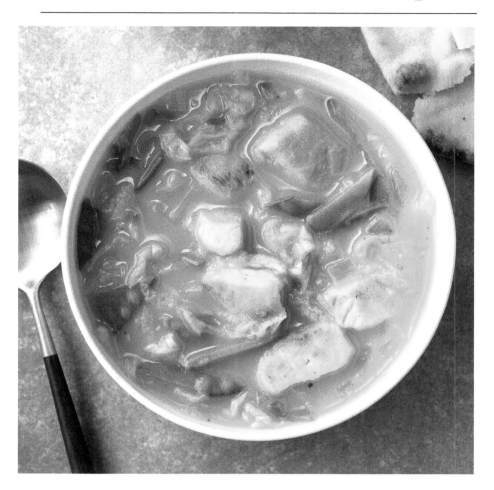

Prep Time: 10 Minutes

Cook Time: 25 Minutes

Total Time: 35 Minutes

Servings: 6 Servings

Ingredients

- 1 1/2 pounds boneless skinless chicken breast, sliced thin
- 1 large onion, peeled and sliced thin
- 1 red bell pepper, quartered and sliced thin
- 1 cup shredded carrots
- 1 cup thinly sliced snap peas
- 1/2 cup roughly chopped Thai basil
- 2 tablespoons vegetable oil
- 1 teaspoon sesame oil
- 1/4 - 1/2 teaspoon crushed red pepper
- 2 tablespoons freshly grated ginger, grated
- 4 cloves garlic, minced
- 64 ounces chicken stock
- 1 1/2 cups unsweetened coconut milk
- 1/4 cup fish sauce
- 1/2 cup chopped green onions for garnish

Instructions

- Place a large saucepot over medium-high heat. Add both oils to the pot, followed by the onions. Saute the onions for 2-3 minutes, stirring regularly. Then add the garlic and ginger and saute for 1 more minute.
- Add the stock, coconut milk, fish sauce, and crushed red pepper. Bring to a boil. Simmer for 10 minutes. Then add the sliced chicken. Stir to separate, then simmer another 5-8 minutes until the chicken is cooked through.
- Turn off the heat and add the red bell peppers, carrots, snap peas, and basil. Cover the pot and steep the vegetable for 5 minutes, until barely cooked through, but still firm. Taste, then salt and pepper as needed. Serve warm with a sprinkle of chopped green onions.

Nutrition

- Calories: 462kcal, Carbohydrates: 22g, Protein: 34g, Fat: 26g, Saturated Fat: 18g, Cholesterol: 81mg, Sodium: 1350mg, Potassium: 1138mg, Fiber: 3g, Sugar: 10g, Vitamin A: 4595iu, Vitamin C: 44mg, Calcium: 60mg, Iron: 2.9mg

15.   Skinny Creamy Chimichurri Chicken Skillet

Prep Time: 5 Minutes

Cook Time: 13 Minutes

Total Time: 18 Minutes

Servings: 4

Ingredients

- 4 boneless skinless chicken breasts
- 1 tablespoon olive oil
- 1 bunch parsley, stems removed
- 1/2 onion, cut into wedges
- 2 cloves garlic
- 3 ounces fat-free cream cheese
- 3 tablespoons red wine vinegar
- 1 tablespoon dried oregano
- 1 1/2 teaspoons ground cumin
- 1/4 teaspoon crushed red pepper
- 1 cup water
- Salt and pepper

Instructions

- Place a large deep skillet over medium heat and add the oil. Season the chicken breasts with salt and pepper. Once the skillet is hot add the chicken breasts and cook 4 minutes per side.
- Meanwhile, peel the onion and garlic cloves. Place the parsley, onion, garlic, vinegar, oregano, cumin, crushed red pepper, and 1/2 teaspoon salt in the food processor. Pulse until the mixture is well chopped. Then add in the cream cheese and water. Turn on and puree until very smooth.
- Once the chicken has seared for 4 minutes per side, pour the sauce over the chicken. Simmer for 3-5 minutes to let the chicken finish

cooking and the sauce thicken. Taste, then salt and pepper as needed.

Nutrition

Calories: 253kcal, Carbohydrates: 4g, Protein: 26g, Fat: 14g, Saturatedfat: 5g, Cholesterol: 95mg, Sodium: 215mg, Potassium: 575mg, Fiber: 1g, Sugar: 1g, Vitamin C: 21.8mg, Calcium: 79mg, Iron: 2.4mg

16.   Chicken Caesar Pasta Salad

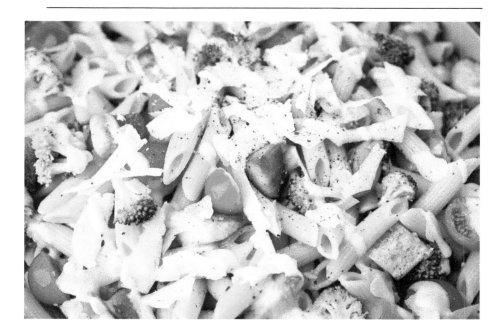

Prep Time: 20 Minutes

Cook Time: 15 Minutes

Total Time: 35 Minutes

Servings: 12

Ingredients

For The Chicken Caesar Pasta Salad:

- 1 1/2 pounds boneless skinless chicken breasts
- 1 pound fusilli pasta
- 1-pint grape tomatoes
- 1 cup pitted black olives
- 1 cup chopped green onions
- 1 head romaine lettuce
- 3/4 cup shredded Parmesan cheese

39

- 2 cups croutons, store-bought or homemade
- Homemade Caesar Dressing
- Salt and pepper

For The Homemade Caesar Dressing:

- 1 cup low-fat buttermilk
- 1/2 cup light mayonnaise
- 1 1/2 tablespoons lemon juice
- 1 tablespoon Dijon mustard
- 7 whole anchovies from a can
- 2 cloves garlic, peeled

Instructions

- Preheat the grill to medium heat. Place a large pot of salted water over high heat and bring to a boil. Salt and pepper the chicken breasts.
- Once the grill is hot, grill the chicken for 5-6 minutes per side. Then remove from heat and allow it to rest. Meanwhile, drop the pasta in the boiling water. Cook for 6-8 minutes, then drain and cool.
- Place all the ingredients for the homemade Caesar dressing in the blender. Puree until smooth. Chop the chicken breasts into bite-size pieces and roughly chop the romaine lettuce.
- To assemble, place the pasta, tomatoes, black olives, and chopped green onions in a large bowl. Top with the chopped grilled chicken Then pour the dressing over the pasta salad and toss to coat. If making ahead, cover the Chicken Caesar Pasta Salad and refrigerate until ready to serve.
- Right before serving, toss in the chopped romaine, shredded Parmesan cheese, and croutons. Salt and pepper to taste. Serve cold or at room temperature.

Nutrition

Calories: 320kcal, Carbohydrates: 39g, Protein: 22g, Fat: 8g, Saturated Fat: 2g, Cholesterol: 44mg, Sodium: 493mg, Potassium: 595mg, Fiber: 4g, Sugar: 4g, Vitamin C: 10.8mg, Calcium: 149mg, Iron: 1.8mg

17.   Bistro Slow Cooker Chicken And Rice

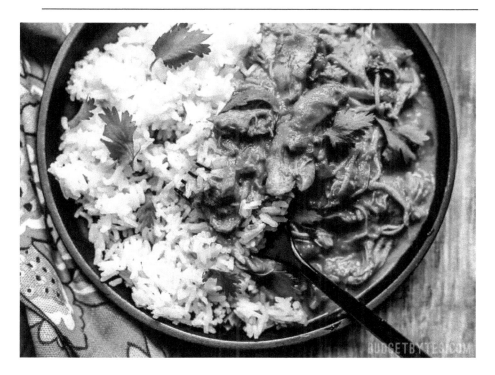

Prep Time: 10 Minutes

Cook Time: 2 Hours

Total Time: 2 Hours 10 Minutes

Servings: 8

Ingredients

- 1 onion, peeled and diced
- 6 cloves garlic, peeled and minced
- 1/4 cup unsalted butter
- 4 boneless skinless chicken breast

- 2 1/2 cups jasmine rice
- Bouquet de garni (bundle of herbs with 2 sprigs of rosemary and 4 sprigs thyme)
- 1 lemon sliced and seeds removed
- 1/2 teaspoon paprika
- 5 cups chicken broth
- Salt
- Pepper

Instructions

- Place the butter in a medium skillet and set over medium heat. Add the chopped onion and garlic. Saute for 3-5 minutes to soften, then pour the onions and butter into the crock of a large slow cooker.
- Add the bouquet de Garni and the chicken to the slow cooker. Sprinkle the chicken with 1 teaspoon salt, 1/2 teaspoon ground pepper, and 1/2 teaspoon paprika. Pour the rice over the top and lay the lemon slices over it. Then pour the chicken broth over the rice.
- Cover and cook on high for 2-3 hours, or on low for 3-5 hours. (The first time you make this dish, be watchful of the rice. All slow cookers are slightly different, and you do not want the rice to cook to mush. Turn the slow cooker off when the rice is firm and fluffy. My slow cooker takes 2 hours on high.)
- Pull the chicken breast and the bouquet de garni out of the crock and cut into bite-size chunks. Add the chicken back to the crock and toss. Serve warm.

Nutrition

Calories: 343kcal, Carbohydrates: 49g, Protein: 17g, Fat: 8g, Saturated Fat: 4g, Cholesterol: 51mg, Sodium: 608mg, Potassium: 422mg, Fiber: 1g, Sugar: 1g, Vitamin C: 13.6mg, Calcium: 37mg, Iron: 1.1mg

18. Sweet and Tangy Chicken Quesadillas

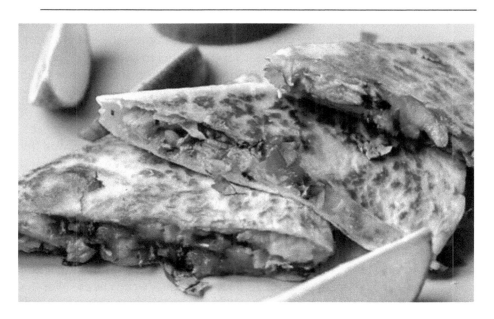

Prep Time: 5 Minutes

Cook Time: 20 Minutes

Total Time: 25 Minutes

Servings: 4 Large Quesadillas

Ingredients

- 1 1/4 pound chicken breast or tenders
- 1 red onion sliced
- 1 orange bell pepper seeded and sliced
- 1 tablespoon butter
- 1/2 cup Musselman's Apple Butter
- 2 tablespoons cayenne pepper sauce
- 4 teaspoons Musselman's Apple Cider Vinegar
- 8 large wheat tortillas

- 3 cups shredded Mexican blend cheese at room temperature
- 1/4 cup chopped cilantro

Instructions

- Preheat a large nonstick skillet to medium-high heat. Chop the chicken into bite-size pieces and set aside. When the skillet is hot, add the sliced onions and sear for 2 minutes to soften and char the edges, flipping once. Move the onions to a plate and sear the sliced peppers for 2 minutes until slightly charred. Move the peppers to the plate as well.
- Add the butter to the skillet. Once melted, add the chicken pieces. Salt and pepper liberally, then brown for 2 minutes per side. Add the apple butter, cayenne pepper sauce, and vinegar. Stir to combine and let the mixture simmer for another 2 minutes. Then turn off the heat and stir to coat the chicken in the sauce. Move the chicken to the holding plate as well.
- Lower the heat to medium-low and add the first tortilla to a clean nonstick skillet. Sprinkle it with a heaping 1/4 cup cheese. Spread one-quarter of the onions, peppers, and chicken over the top. Then sprinkle with fresh cilantro. Sprinkle another 1/4 cup cheese over the top and cover with a second tortilla.
- Wait to flip the quesadilla until the bottom tortilla is golden brown, and the cheese has started to melt to hold everything together. Place a flat spatula under the bottom tortilla, and another on the top tortilla. Then quickly flip the quesadilla. Brown the bottom tortilla, then move to a warming drawer or warm oven to keep crisp. Repeat with the remaining ingredients. Once all 4 quesadillas of cooked, cut them into wedges and serve warm!

Nutrition

Calories: 1170kcal, Carbohydrates: 67g, Protein: 81g, Fat: 63g, Saturatedfat: 35g, Cholesterol: 267mg, Sodium: 2235mg, Potassium: 810mg, Fiber: 8g, Sugar: 21g, Vitamin C: 42.2mg, Calcium: 1351mg, Iron: 4.1mg

19.   Korean Fried Chicken Recipe

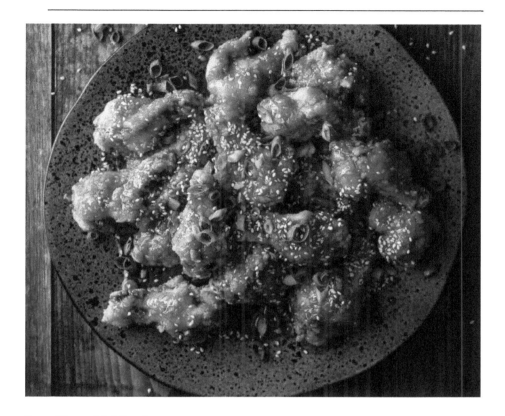

Prep Time: 10 Minutes

Cook Time: 30 Minutes

Resting Time: 4 Hours

Total Time: 4 Hours 40 Minutes

Servings: 12

Ingredients

- For the Fried Chicken Recipe
- 4 pounds whole chicken, wings, and drumsticks about 12 pieces
- 1/2 cup salt + 1-quart warm water

- 1 1/4 cup corn starch divided
- 1 tablespoon baking powder divided
- 3/4 cup all-purpose flour
- 12-ounce light beer or club soda
- 2 quarts fry oil peanut, canola, grape seed
- For the Korean Dunking Sauce
- 1/2 cup gochujang sauce
- 1/4 cup low-sodium soy sauce
- 1/4 cup rice vinegar
- 1/4 cup brown sugar
- 3 tablespoons sesame oil
- 5 cloves garlic smashed
- 1 tablespoon fresh grated ginger
- 1-2 tablespoons Sriracha optional for extra heat

Instructions

- Place the salt and warm water in a large bowl and swirl to dissolve the salt. Then add the chicken pieces to the brine. Cover and refrigerate for 4 hours (or up to 12 hours.) Take the chicken out of the brine and dry with paper towels. Set out to allow the skin to continue drying.
- Pour the oil into a large heavy-bottomed stockpot and set over medium heat. Attach a deep-fry thermometer if you have one. Mix 3/4 cup of cornstarch and 2 teaspoons of baking powder in a bowl. Move the chicken to the bowl and toss to coat well.
- Then place the remaining 1/2 cup of cornstarch, 1 teaspoon baking powder, and 3/4 cup of flour in a separate bowl. Whisk in the beer to create the tempura batter.
- Turn the oven on warm (175-200 degrees F) and set out an oven-safe plate lined with paper towels. Check the temperature of the frying oil. It should be at 350 degrees F. Drop a little batter into the oil to check. If the batter turns brown right away the oil is too hot. Turn off the heat and wait for it to cool, before continuing. One-piece at a time, tap the excess cornstarch off the chicken and dunk it in the tempura batter. Dunk a couple of times to make sure there are no air pockets. Shake the chicken a little to allow the excess batter to drip back into the bowl then slowly swirl the chicken as you place it in the oil. Continue... frying 4-6 pieces at a time, until golden brown and

46

Servings: 20 Tacos

Ingredients

For The Vietnamese Banh Mi Chicken

- 2 tablespoons coconut oil
- 2 pounds boneless skinless chicken thighs
- 1/2 cup fresh lime juice
- 1/3 cup fish sauce
- 1/4 cup granulated sugar
- 1 jalapeno
- 4 cloves garlic minced

- For The Spicy Mayo
- 3/4 cup mayonnaise
- 1-2 tablespoons Sriracha
- 1 tablespoon rice vinegar
- 1 tablespoon granulated sugar
- For the Street Tacos
- 2 packages Old El Paso Flour Tortillas taco size
- 3 carrots shredded
- 1 English cucumber sliced thin
- 2 bunches radishes sliced thin
- 4 jalapenos sliced
- 1 bunch fresh mint or cilantro
- 2 limes cut into wedges

Instructions

For The Vietnamese Banh Mi Chicken:

- Pour the fish sauce, lime juice, and sugar into a medium microwave-safe bowl. Microwave for 1-2 minutes, until the sugar dissolves. Cut the chicken thighs into very small (1/-inch) pieces. Place in a bowl along with jalapeno slices and minced garlic. Stir and refrigerate for at least 1 hour. (3 hours is best!)

For The Spicy Mayo:

- Place the rice vinegar and sugar in a small microwave-safe bowl. Microwave for 1 minute to dissolve the sugar. Then mix in the mayo and Sriracha. Add more Sriracha for an extra kick. Refrigerate until ready to serve.
- Prep all the veggies. Once the chicken has marinated, drain off the marinade. Then heat a large skillet to medium-high heat. Once hot, add 1 tablespoon coconut oil to the skillet. Then add half the chicken to the skillet. Sear for 4-5 minutes, stirring to caramelize on all sides. Remove and repeat with the remaining chicken.

To Serve:

- Place a scoop of chicken in Old El Paso flour tortillas. Top with shredded carrots, cucumber slices, radishes, fresh mint leaves, and jalapeno slices. Drizzle with spicy mayo and serve with fresh lime wedges.

Nutrition

Calories: 234kcal, Carbohydrates: 21g, Protein: 12g, Fat: 12g, Saturated Fat: 3g, Cholesterol: 47mg, Sodium: 618mg, Potassium: 250mg, Fiber: 1g, Sugar: 6g, Vitamin C: 10.4mg, Calcium: 47mg, Iron: 1.5mg

22.   Asian Chicken Sliders With Slaw

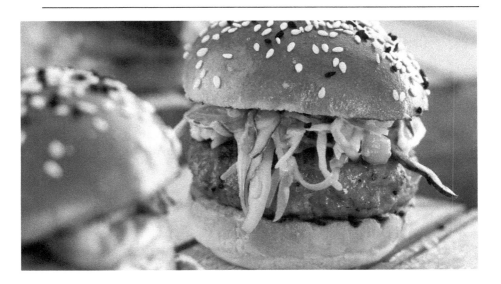

Prep Time: 15 Minutes

Cook Time: 6 Minutes

Total Time: 21 Minutes

Servings: 12

Ingredients

For The Asian Chicken Sliders:

- 1 pound ground chicken, or ground white meat turkey
- 1/2 cup jasmine rice, cooked
- 1/4 cup panko bread crumbs
- 1/4 cup chopped green onions
- 1 jalapeno, seeded and diced
- 1 tablespoon grated ginger
- 1 large egg
- 4 tablespoons Bertolli 100% Pure Olive Oil, divided
- 2 tablespoons soy sauce

- 12 small yeast buns, dinner rolls
- 1/2 cup wasabi mayonnaise (1/2 cup mayo + 1 teaspoon wasabi paste)

For The Asian Slaw:

- 2 cups shredded napa cabbage
- 1/2 cup shredded carrots
- 1/2 cup mung bean sprouts
- 1/2 ripe mango, cut julienne
- 1/4 cup chopped cilantro
- 3 tablespoons rice vinegar
- 2 tablespoon Bertolli Extra Virgin Olive Oil
- Salt and pepper

Instructions

- Preheat the grill to medium heat, approximately 350 degrees F. Place the ground chicken, jasmine rice, panko, green onions, jalapeno, and ginger in a large bowl. Crack the egg into the bowl and add 1 tablespoon Bertolli® 100% Pure Olive Oil, and soy sauce. Mix the ingredients by hand until well combined.
- Scoop 3 tablespoon portions of chicken mixture and roll into tight balls. Place on a foil-lined baking sheet. Press the balls flat with the back of a spatula, to 1/2 inch thick. Brush the tops with olive oil.
- Cut the rolls in half and brush the insides with Bertolli 100% Pure Olive Oil.

For The Asian Slaw:

- Mix the napa cabbage, carrots, mung bean sprouts, mango, and cilantro in a medium bowl. Drizzle with rice vinegar and Bertolli® Extra Virgin Olive Oil. Toss to coat, then season with salt and pepper to taste.
- Grill the buns for 1 minute. Remove from the grill. Then place the chicken patties on the grill top-side-down and grill for 2 minutes. Brush the tops of the patties with oil. Flip, and grill another 2-3 minutes.

To Assemble:

- Smear the buns with wasabi mayo. Then add the chicken patties, and top with Asian slaw. Place the bun topper on the slaw and serve!

Nutrition

Calories: 356kcal, Carbohydrates: 45g, Protein: 14g, Fat: 12g, Saturated Fat: 2g, Cholesterol: 46mg, Sodium: 506mg, Potassium: 345mg, Fiber: 2g, Sugar: 7g, Vitamin C: 16.2mg, Calcium: 37mg, Iron: 11.5mg

23.   Jamaican Jerk Chicken Thighs

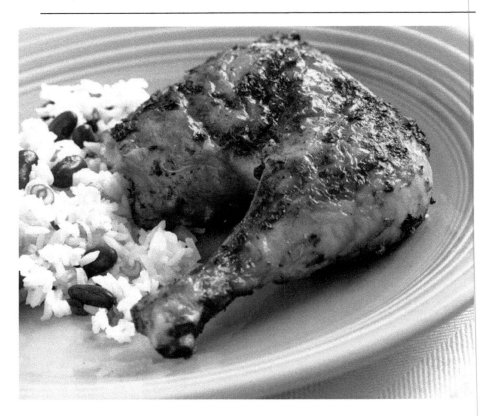

Prep Time: 10 Minutes

Cook Time: 15 Minutes

Total Time: 25 Minutes

Servings: 8

Ingredients

- 4-4.5 pounds boneless skinless chicken thighs
- 1 bunch scallions, trimmed and cut into chunks
- 6 garlic cloves, peeled
- 3-4 habanero peppers, stemmed and seeded

- 1 piece fresh ginger (2-inch piece)
- 1/4 cup fresh lime juice + zest of 3 limes
- 1/4 cup olive oil
- 3 tablespoons soy sauce
- 3 tablespoons brown sugar
- 1 tablespoon salt
- 1 tablespoon dried thyme
- 1 tablespoon allspice
- 1 teaspoon ground black pepper
- 1 teaspoon ground nutmeg
- 1 teaspoon ground cinnamon

Instructions

- Place the chicken thighs in a large gallon zip bag. Place all remaining ingredients in the food processor. Puree on high until well-combined and pasty.
- Pour the jerk marinade over the chicken in the zip bag. Close the bag tightly and gently massage the bag to ensure all the chicken thighs are coated in marinade. Refrigerate for 3 to 48 hours. (The longer the marinade time, the more complex and spicy the chicken will taste.)
- Preheat the grill to medium heat, approximately 350-400 degrees F. Once hot, carefully brush the grates with oil. Take the chicken out of the bag with tongs and grill for 5-7 minutes per side. Serve warm!

Nutrition

Calories: 168kcal, Carbohydrates: 9g, Protein: 12g, Fat: 9g, Saturated Fat: 1g, Cholesterol: 53mg, Sodium: 1303mg, Potassium: 260mg, Fiber: 1g, Sugar: 5g, Vitamin C: 37.4mg, Calcium: 36mg, Iron: 1.6mg

24.   Thai Chicken Noodle Bowl With Peanut Sauce

Prep Time: 15 Minutes

Cook Time: 20 Minutes

Total Time: 35 Minutes

Servings: 6

Ingredients

For The Thai Chicken Noodle Bowl:

- 1 pound boneless skinless chicken breast 2 large
- 1 tablespoon fresh grated ginger
- 2 cloves garlic minced
- 1/4 cup fish sauce
- 1/4 cup soy sauce
- 1 tablespoon sesame oil
- 1 tablespoon chile-garlic sauce
- 1 pound DeLallo Whole Wheat Capellini Pasta
- 6 ounces mung bean sprouts
- 1 cup fresh basil leaves use Thai Basil if you can find it
- 3/4 cup sliced green onions
- 1 cup sliced cucumber
- 1/2 cup roasted peanuts
- 2 limes cut into wedges

For The Peanut Sauce:

- 1/2 cup peanut butter
- 1 tablespoon fresh grated ginger
- 1/3 cup chicken broth
- 1 tablespoon honey
- 1/4 cup soy sauce
- 3 tablespoons rice vinegar

- 3 tablespoons sesame oil
- 2 cloves garlic
- 1 tablespoon chile-garlic sauce optional

Instructions

- Place the chicken in a baking dish and top with grated ginger, garlic, fish sauce, soy sauce, sesame oil, and chile-garlic sauce. Allow the chicken to soak while you prep the rest of the ingredients.
- Preheat the grill to medium heat and bring a large pot of water to boil. Meanwhile, place all the ingredients for the peanut sauce in the blender. Puree until smooth.
- Grill the chicken for approximately 5 minutes per side, then place on a plate and cover with foil to keep warm.
- Drop the pasta in the boiling water, cook according to package instructions (about 2-3 minutes) then drain.
- After the chicken has rested for at least 5 minutes, slice it into pieces. Then toss the pasta with the peanut sauce and divide into bowls. Top each bowl with chicken slices, bean sprouts, basil leaves, green onion, cucumber slices, peanuts, and a couple of lime wedges.

Nutrition

Calories: 691kcal, Carbohydrates: 75g, Protein: 40g, Fat: 29g, Saturated Fat: 5g, Cholesterol: 48mg, Sodium: 2416mg, Potassium: 897mg, Fiber: 4g, Sugar: 9g, Vitamin C: 16.5mg, Calcium: 97mg, Iron: 5mg

25. Chicken Marsala Recipe With Tomatoes And Basil

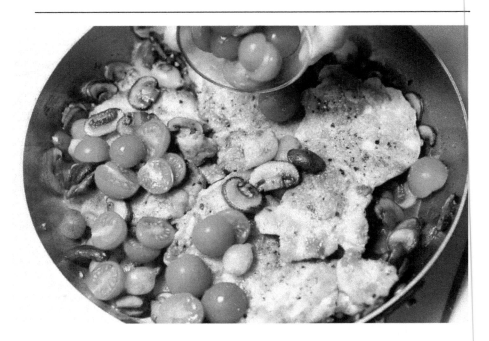

Prep Time: 15 Minutes

Cook Time: 25 Minutes

Total Time: 40 Minutes

Servings: 4

Ingredients

- 2 large boneless skinless chicken breasts or 6 chicken cutlets
- 1/4 cup all-purpose flour could be a gluten-free baking mix
- 1 tablespoon butter
- 1 tablespoon olive oil
- 1-pint cherry tomatoes
- 1 shallot peeled and sliced
- 3 cloves garlic peeled and minced

- 1 pound cremini mushrooms sliced thin
- 1/2 cup marsala wine
- 1/4 cup chicken broth
- 1/4 cup fresh chopped parsley
- 1/4 cup fresh basil leaves
- Parmesan cheese for garnish

Instructions

- If working with whole chicken breasts, slice each one into 3 flat cutlets. Place them on a cutting board and cover with plastic wrap. Use a meat tenderizer (or rolling pin) to beat the chicken cutlets into thin even pieces. Place the flour in a shallow dish and season with 1 teaspoon salt and 1/2 teaspoon ground pepper. Then coat the chicken cutlets in flour and dust off.
- Heat a large skillet over medium-high heat. Add 1/2 tablespoon butter and 1/2 tablespoon oil to the skillet. Once melted, add 3 cutlets to the skillet at a time, cooking for 2-3 minutes per side. Remove and cover with foil. Then repeat with the remaining cutlets.
- Add the tomatoes to the skillet and let them blister on several sides, swirling the pan a few times. Once the first tomato pops, remove it from the skillet and cover it with foil.
- Add the remaining butter and oil to the skillet. Then add the mushrooms, shallots, and garlic. Saute the mushrooms until they are soft. Then add the marsala wine and broth. Cook until most of the liquid is absorbed. Add the chicken and tomatoes back to the skillet and toss. Turn off the heat and toss in the fresh basil leaves and parsley. Serve warm with parmesan cheese, if desired.

Nutrition

Calories: 253kcal, Carbohydrates: 22g, Protein: 17g, Fat: 8g, Saturated Fat: 3g, Cholesterol: 44mg, Sodium: 170mg, Potassium: 1065mg, Fiber: 2g, Sugar: 8g, Vitamin C: 35.1mg, Calcium: 48mg, Iron: 2.3mg

26.   280. Chicken Broccoli Slow Cooker Lasagna

Prep Time: 15 Minutes

Cook Time: 3 Hours

Total Time: 3 Hours 15 Minutes

Servings: 8

Ingredients

- 1 box DeLallo No-Boil Lasagna Noodles
- 2 packages of cream cheese (8-ounce packages) could be low fat
- 1/2 cup diced onion
- 2 cloves garlic minced
- 1 cup milk
- 4 cups small broccoli florets
- 1 1/4 pounds boneless skinless chicken breast
- 4 cups shredded sharp cheddar cheese
- Salt and pepper

Instructions

- Spray a large slow cooker with nonstick cooking spray. Place the cream cheese, onions, and garlic in a microwave-safe bowl with 1 teaspoon salt, and 1/4 teaspoon ground pepper. Microwave on high for 1-2 minutes, until the cream cheese, is molten and the onions are soft. Pour in the milk and whisk until smooth.
- Cut the broccoli into small florets and slice the chicken into small bite-size pieces.
- Spread a small amount of the cream cheese sauce in the bottom of the slow cooker. Then cover it with a single layer of dried lasagna sheets. Break the noodles to fit into the slow cooker along the round edges. Sprinkle the pasta sheets with 1 cup of broccoli, one-quarter of the chopped chicken, and 1 cup of shredded cheese. Drizzle one-quarter of the remaining cream cheese sauce over the ingredients.

Repeat the lasagna sheet, chicken, broccoli, cheese, and sauce layering until you have 4 full layers.

- Place the crock in the slow cooker and cover with the lid. Slow cooker for 2-3 hours on high, or 4-6 hours on low. Cut and serve warm.

Nutrition

Calories: 670kcal, Carbohydrates: 53g, Protein: 43g, Fat: 31g, Saturated Fat: 18g, Cholesterol: 138mg, Sodium: 731mg, Potassium: 781mg, Fiber: 3g, Sugar: 8g, Vitamin C: 42.4mg, Calcium: 566mg, Iron: 1.8mg

27.   Nam Sod Lettuce Wraps

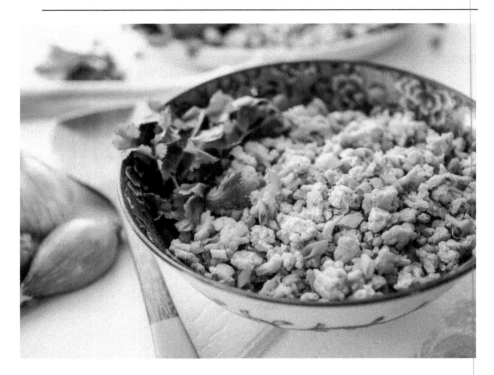

Prep Time: 20 Minutes

Cook Time: 8 Minutes

Total Time: 28 Minutes

Servings: 4

Ingredients

- 1 teaspoon peanut oil
- 1 pound ground pork
- 2 cloves garlic minced
- 1 tablespoon fresh ginger grated
- 1 tablespoon fresh mint chopped
- 2 teaspoons low sodium soy sauce

- 1 tablespoon fish sauce
- 2 tablespoon lime juice
- 1/4 teaspoon crushed red pepper
- 1 head butter lettuce leaves separated
- 1 cup shredded carrot
- 1 cup sliced red onion
- 1 cup chopped green onions scallions
- 1 cup chopped cilantro
- 1 cup dry roasted peanuts
- 1 cup sliced red bell pepper optional

Instructions

- Place a large skillet over medium heat. Add the oil, ground pork, garlic, and ginger. Brown for 5 minutes, breaking into small pieces with a wooden spoon. Then add the mint, soy sauce, fish sauce, lime juice, and crushed red pepper. Stir and cook for another 3 minutes until the liquid absorbs.
- For Lettuce Wraps: Place a spoonful of the Nam sod meat filling in lettuce leaves, then top with veggies and peanuts.
- For The Salad: Arrange the lettuce leaves in 4 serving bowls, then divide the nam sod between the bowls and top with veggies and peanuts.

Nutrition

Calories: 591kcal, Carbohydrates: 22g, Protein: 31g, Fat: 44g, Saturated Fat: 12g, Cholesterol: 82mg, Sodium: 791mg, Potassium: 1011mg, Fiber: 7g, Sugar: 8g, Vitamin C: 63.6mg, Calcium: 99mg, Iron: 3.2mg

28. Southwest Chicken Caesar Salad

Prep Time: 20 Minutes

Cook Time: 30 Minutes

Total Time: 50 Minutes

Servings: 6

Ingredients

- 1 1/2 pounds new small potatoes halved
- 1 1/2 pounds chicken tenders
- 5-6 ounces fresh chopped romaine or green leaf lettuce
- 2 avocados sliced
- 3 corn cobs corn cut off
- 1 poblano pepper seeded and chopped
- 1 cup dried cherries
- 1 shallot peeled and diced
- 1 clove garlic minced
- 1 tablespoon butter
- 2 tablespoons olive oil divided
- Newman's Own Creamy Caesar Dressing
- Salt and pepper

Instructions

- Preheat the oven to 450 degrees F. Cut the potatoes in half, lengthwise, and place on a rimmed baking sheet. Drizzle with 1 tablespoon olive oil, toss, and sprinkle with salt and pepper. Bake for 30 minutes, flipping once.
- Preheat the grill (or a grill pan) to medium heat. Drizzle the remaining olive oil over the chicken tenders. Salt and pepper and toss to coat. Grill the chicken for 4-5 minutes per side, then set aside.
- Place the butter in a large skillet. Once melted, add the chopped shallots, garlic, and poblano peppers. Saute for 2-3 minutes, then add the corn. Saute another 4-5 minutes, then toss in the cherries and salt and pepper to taste. Remove from heat.

- To serve, pile the lettuce in a large serving bowl (or on individual dinner plates.) Cut the chicken into bite-size pieces. Then top the greens with roasted potatoes, sliced avocado, and grilled chicken. Spoon the corn salsa over the top, and drizzle with Newman's Own Creamy Caesar Dressing.

Nutrition

Calories: 523kcal, Carbohydrates: 51g, Protein: 31g, Fat: 23g, Saturated Fat: 5g, Cholesterol: 80mg, Sodium: 232mg, Potassium: 1450mg, Fiber: 11g, Sugar: 16g, Vitamin C: 50.8mg, Calcium: 58mg, Iron: 2.6mg

29.   **Best Chicken Pot Pie Recipe**

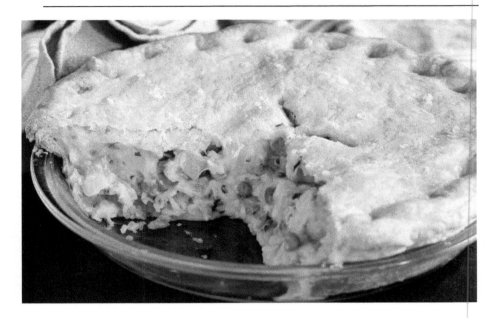

Prep Time: 20 Minutes

Cook Time: 40 Minutes

Total Time: 1 Hour

Servings: 4 Mini Pot Pies

Ingredients

- 1 cup all-purpose flour
- 1 teaspoon sugar
- 1/2 teaspoon salt
- 1/2 cup Land O Lakes Unsalted Butter COLD
- 3 tablespoons ice-cold water more as needed
- For the Pot Pie Recipe:
- 8 ounces chicken tenders cut into bite-size pieces
- 1/4 cup chopped onion
- 1 garlic clove minced

- 1 tablespoon Land O Lakes® Unsalted Butter
- 2 teaspoons all-purpose flour
- 1 teaspoon fresh thyme leaves
- 2 teaspoons chopped parsley
- 1-2 dashes of cayenne pepper
- 3/4 teaspoon chicken base or 1 bouillon cube
- 3/4 cup water
- 3 tablespoon heavy cream
- 3/4 cup frozen peas and carrots mix
- Egg wash 1 egg + 1 tablespoon water, whisked
- Salt and pepper

Instructions

- For the pastry dough, place the flour, sugar, and salt in the food processor and pulse a few times. Pour water over a cup of ice to chill. Then cut the cold butter into cubes and add to the flour. Pulse several times until the butter is cut into the size of peas. Add 3 tablespoons of ice water (without the ice) and pulse again until the dough absorbs the flour and looks like soft pebbles.
- Flour a work surface and dump the crumbly dough out onto the surface. Press together into a flat square, then fold toward the center into a 3-section fold. Roll the dough down to 3/4 inch and fold again in the same manner. If the dough is not coming together, sprinkle 1 teaspoon of ice water over the top and keep folding. Fold and roll the dough 3-4 times, until it is smooth. Then fold into a rectangle, wrap in plastic, and chill.
- Preheat the oven to 400o F and spray a muffin tin (or four 6-ounce ramekins) with non-stick cooking spray. Place a large skillet over medium heat and add the butter and onions. Sauté 2 minutes, then add the chicken pieces and garlic. Sauté for another 2-3 minutes, then add the flour, herbs, and chicken base. Stir to coat. Pour in the water and cream, then stir well. Allow the mixture to come to a simmer to thicken, then add the frozen veggies. Taste for salt and pepper and add a couple of dashes of cayenne for a little kick. Remove from heat.
- Now take the pastry dough out of the fridge and roll it out into a 12-inch circle/square. Cut it into 4 equal triangular pieces. Then fit each piece down into the prepared muffin tin. Spread them apart—they grow! Fill the pastry dough with chicken filling, spooning in the

creamy base. Then loosely fold the flaps over the top. It's okay if there are gaps in the top as long as the pastry dough sides come up high. Brush the egg wash over the top of the pastry dough. Bake for 20-25 minutes on the bottom rack, until golden brown. Allow them to cool for 10 minutes.

- To serve, run a butter knife around the inside edge of the muffin tins. Tip the knife down and carefully lift each pot pie out. If you accidentally poke a hole in the pot pie, serve it in a bowl.

Nutrition

Calories: 475kcal, Carbohydrates: 30g, Protein: 17g, Fat: 32g, Saturated Fat: 19g, Cholesterol: 120mg, Sodium: 479mg, Potassium: 309mg, Fiber: 2g, Sugar: 2g, Vitamin C: 5.4mg, Calcium: 29mg, Iron: 2.1mg

30.   Chicken Salad Recipe With Berries

Prep Time: 15 Minutes

Total Time: 15 Minutes

Servings: 6

Ingredients

- 1 whole rotisserie or baked chicken boned and shredded into chunks
- 1/2 cup light mayonnaise
- 1 teaspoon Dijon mustard
- 4 ounces NatureBox Cherry Berry Bonanza dried cherries, blueberries, and cranberries
- 1/2 cup toasted sliced almonds
- 3/4 cup chopped celery
- 1/2 cup chopped green onion
- Salt and pepper to taste

Instructions

- Chop the celery and green onions and add all the ingredients to a large bowl.
- Stir to thoroughly coat, then salt and pepper to taste. Keep in an air-tight container in the fridge until ready to serve.

Nutrition

Calories: 451kcal, Carbohydrates: 19g, Protein: 28g, Fat: 29g, Saturated Fat: 7g, Cholesterol: 98mg, Sodium: 252mg, Potassium: 380mg, Fiber: 4g, Sugar: 11g, Vitamin C: 4mg, Calcium: 74mg, Iron: 2mg

31.   Spicy Oven Chicken Wings With Apple Onion Dip

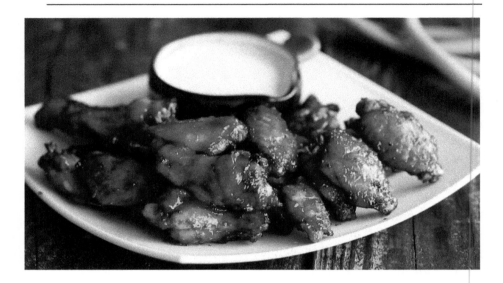

Prep Time: 10 Minutes

Cook Time: 50 Minutes

Total Time: 1 Hour

Servings: 6

Ingredients

For The Spicy Oven Chicken Wings:

- 3 pounds chicken wings or drumettes
- 3 tablespoons vegetable oil
- 1 teaspoon garlic powder
- 1/4 cup Dijon mustard
- 1/4 cup spicy whole-grain mustard-like Lusty Monk
- 1/4 cup maple syrup or honey
- 1 tablespoon Sriracha chili sauce

For The Apple Onion Dip:

- 1 tablespoon butter
- 1 small onion diced
- 3 tablespoons Musselman's Apple Butter
- 1 cup plain Greek yogurt
- 1 tablespoon Dijon mustard
- 1 teaspoon Musselman's Apple Cider Vinegar
- Salt and pepper

Instructions

- Preheat the oven to 450 degrees F and line a large rimmed baking sheet with foil. Dry the chicken wings thoroughly with paper towels, then toss with oil, garlic powder, 1 1/2 teaspoons salt, and 1/2 teaspoon pepper. Spread evenly over the baking sheet. Bake the wings for 20 minutes. Flip, then bake another 15-20 minutes until the skin is crisp.
- Meanwhile, whisk the mustards, maple syrup, and Sriracha together. Once the chicken has cooked through and the skin is crispy, pour the sauce over the chicken and toss to coat. Spread the wings back out and bake another 10 minutes.

For The Apple Onion Dip:

- While the chicken is baking, place a small skillet of medium-low heat. Add the butter and onions and saute for 10-15 minutes until the onions are caramelized.
- Mix the onions with the Musselman's apple butter, Greek yogurt, dijon, and Musselman's apple cider vinegar. Salt and pepper to taste. Serve the spicy chicken wings warm, with the apple onion dip.

Nutrition

Calories: 445kcal, Carbohydrates: 17g, Protein: 27g, Fat: 30g, Saturated Fat: 13g, Cholesterol: 101mg, Sodium: 443mg, Potassium: 337mg, Fiber: 1g, Sugar: 13g, Vitamin C: 4.1mg, Calcium: 82mg, Iron: 1.5mg

32.   Chai Pani's Malabar Chicken Curry

Prep Time: 15 Minutes

Cook Time: 1 Hour

Total Time: 1 Hour 15 Minutes

Servings: 4

Ingredients

- 2 pounds chicken breast cut into bite-size pieces
- 1/2 cup vegetable oil + 1 tablespoon
- 1 1/2 teaspoons mustard seeds
- 1/2 teaspoon fenugreek seeds
- 12-15 curry leaves finely chopped
- 2-3 small dried red chiles cayenne, bird...
- 4 cups chopped red onion about 2 large onions
- 2 1/2 tablespoons grated ginger
- 1 teaspoon chili powder
- 1 1/2 tablespoons ground coriander
- 1 teaspoon turmeric
- 1/2 cup chopped cilantro leaves and/or stems
- 3 cups chopped tomatoes
- 2 tablespoons fresh lime juice
- 1 teaspoon salt
- 1 cup unsweetened coconut milk

Instructions

- Pour 1/2 cup oil in a large saucepot over medium heat. When the oil is hot, add the mustard seeds, fenugreek seeds, curry leaves, and red chiles.
- Sauté for 1-2 minutes, then add the ginger and onions. Reduce the heat to medium-low and allow the onions to brown until they are dark and soft enough the smash with a spatula about 25-30 minutes.

- Add the chili powder, coriander, turmeric, and cilantro mix.
- Raise the heat back to medium and add the tomatoes, salt, and lime juice. Simmer, stirring occasionally, until the tomatoes have disintegrated and the oil separates 15-20 minutes.
- Add 1/2 cup of water and 1 cup coconut milk. Bring to a boil, then turn down the heat.
- In a separate skillet, heat 1 tablespoon of oil over high. Add the chicken to the skillet and brown on all sides, leaving the centers pink 2-4 minutes.
- Add the chicken to the curry and simmer for 5-7 minutes until the chicken has cooked through. Serve over basmati rice.

Nutrition

Calories: 750kcal, Carbohydrates: 30g, Protein: 54g, Fat: 49g, Saturated Fat: 36g, Cholesterol: 145mg, Sodium: 1129mg, Potassium: 1644mg, Fiber: 7g, Sugar: 14g, Vitamin A: 740iu, Vitamin C: 96.4mg, Calcium: 142mg, Iron: 4.8mg

33. Ethiopian Recipes: Doro Wat And Injera Recipe

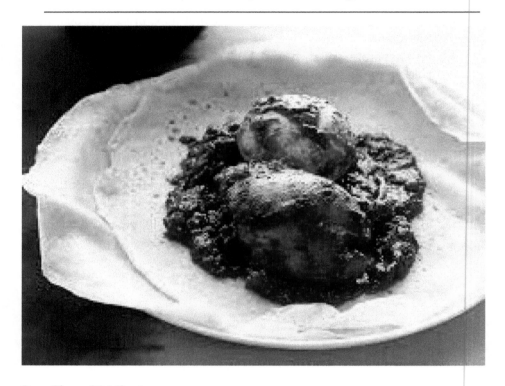

Prep Time: 30 Minutes

Cook Time: 6 Minutes

Total Time: 36 Minutes

Servings: 8

Ingredients

For The Doro Wat:

- 3 pounds boneless chicken breasts and thighs, cut into 1-inch cubes
- 2 large onions chopped

- 4 cloves garlic minced
- 1 cup butter
- 1 cup red wine
- 2 cups water
- 2 teaspoons salt
- 1 teaspoon ground cardamom
- 2 tablespoons garam masala
- 1/3 cup hot smoked paprika
- 1 tablespoon crushed red pepper
- 2 teaspoons fenugreek seeds
- 1 tablespoon dried thyme
- 3 tablespoons tomato paste
- 1 tablespoon sugar
- 1 lime juiced
- For the Injera Recipe:
- 3 cups all-purpose flour
- 1 cup buckwheat flour
- 2 tablespoons baking soda
- 1 teaspoon salt
- 4 cups club soda
- 1 cup white vinegar or rice vinegar
- Oil for pan

Instructions

For The Doro Wat:

- Place all the ingredients, minus the lime juice, in a slow cooker and cover. Cook for 4-6 hours depending on your slow cooker settings until the chicken is tender. Then mash the chicken to shreds with a potato masher (or the bottom of a ladle.) Stir in the lime juice and keep warm.
- For the Injera Recipe:
- In a large bowl, mix both flours, salt, and baking soda. Whisk in the club soda until smooth. Then add the vinegar and whisk.
- Heat a large skillet over medium heat. Pour oil on a paper towel and wipe the skillet with the oiled paper towel.

- Using a scoop, pour batter into the skillet creating a 6-inch circle. Carefully swirl the pan around to thin out the batter until it measures 8- to 9-inches across.
- Cook for 1 minute, then using a large spatula, flip the Injera over and cook another minute. Remove from the skillet and stack on a plate. Repeat with the remaining batter. The Injera will seem slightly crisp in the pan but will soften immediately when placed on the plate.
- Once finished cooking the Injera. Cut the circles in half with a pizza cutter, roll into tubes, and stack. Keep warm until ready to serve. Serve the Doro Wat and Injera together, tearing a piece of Injera and using it to pick up the Doro Wat.

Nutrition

Calories: 705kcal, Carbohydrates: 59g, Protein: 45g, Fat: 30g, Saturated Fat: 16g, Cholesterol: 170mg, Sodium: 2233mg, Potassium: 1078mg, Fiber: 7g, Sugar: 5g, Vitamin A: 3635iu, Vitamin C: 8.6mg, Calcium: 88mg, Iron: 6.1mg

34. Cool Chicken Taco Pasta Salad

Prep Time: 15 Minutes

Cook Time: 10 Minutes

Total Time: 25 Minutes

Servings: 8

Ingredients

- 1 pound fusilli pasta
- 3 cups chopped cooked chicken, leftover or rotisserie
- 1-pint cherry tomatoes halved
- 1 cup chopped scallions
- 3.8 ounces sliced black olives (1 can)
- 1/4 cup chopped cilantro
- 8 ounces French or Catalina Dressing (1 bottle)
- 1/2 cup sour cream
- 1 packet Old El Paso Taco Seasoning
- 4.5 ounce Old El Paso Chopped Green Chiles (1 can)
- 1/2 cup shredded Mexican blend cheese (optional)

Instructions

- Boil a large pot of water and cook the fusilli pasta according to package instructions. Drain and rinse under cold water to cook the pasta. Shake off excess water and pour the pasta into a large salad bowl.
- Add the chopped chicken, tomatoes, scallions, black olives, and cilantro to the pasta.
- In a separate bowl, combine the French dressing with sour cream, Old El Paso Taco Seasoning, and Chopped Green Chiles. Stir until smooth.
- Pour the dressing over the pasta salad and toss well to coat. Toss in the shredded cheese if desired. Cover and chill until ready to serve.

Nutrition

Calories: 529kcal, Carbohydrates: 54g, Protein: 18g, Fat: 26g, Saturated Fat: 6g, Cholesterol: 45mg, Sodium: 964mg, Potassium: 438mg, Fiber: 4g, Sugar: 9g, Vitamin C: 25.2mg, Calcium: 114mg, Iron: 2.6mg

35. Bruschetta Chicken Sheet Pan Dinner

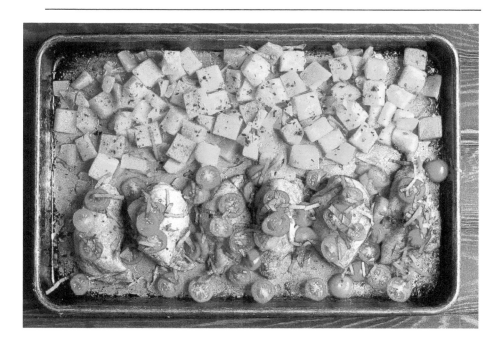

Prep Time: 12 Minutes

Cook Time: 18 Minutes

Total Time: 30 Minutes

Servings: 4

Ingredients

- 2 large boneless skinless chicken breasts
- 3 tablespoon olive oil, divided
- 3/4 teaspoon dried Italian seasoning, divided
- 1 pound asparagus, trimmed
- 8-ounce fresh mozzarella ball
- 12 ounces grape tomatoes, mixed colors

- 2 cloves garlic minced
- 8-10 leaves fresh basil, chopped
- 2 teaspoon balsamic vinegar, divided
- Salt and pepper

Instructions

- Preheat the oven to 400 degrees F. Line a large rimmed sheet pan with parchment paper. Lay each chicken breast flat and cut in half, parallel to the cutting board, to make four thinner chicken breasts. Rub each piece with olive oil and sprinkle both sides with 1/2 teaspoon Italian seasoning. Then salt and pepper liberally. Place the chicken breasts in a line down one long edge of the sheet pan. Bake for 10 minutes.
- Meanwhile, slice the mozzarella ball into four equal rounds. Then cut the grape tomatoes into quarters and place them in a bowl. Add the garlic, chopped basil, 2 tablespoons olive oil, and 1 teaspoon balsamic vinegar. Toss well, then season with salt and pepper to taste.
- After 10 minutes, take the sheet pan out of the oven. Flip the chicken breasts over and place one slice of mozzarella over each chicken breast. Then spread the asparagus out on the empty side of the sheet pan. Drizzle the asparagus with 1/2 tablespoon olive oil, 1 teaspoon balsamic vinegar, 1/4 teaspoon Italian seasoning, salt, and pepper.
- Place the sheet pan back in the oven and bake for another 8-10 minutes. Remove from the oven and top the chicken with the tomatoes bruschetta salad. Serve the bruschetta chicken with a side of roasted asparagus.

Nutrition

Calories: 370kcal, Carbohydrates: 10g, Protein: 27g, Fat: 24g, Saturated Fat: 9g, Cholesterol: 80mg, Sodium: 428mg, Potassium: 682mg, Fiber: 3g, Sugar: 5g, Vitamin A: 2020iu, Vitamin C: 19.1mg, Calcium: 334mg, Iron: 3.3mg

36. Yakhni Pulao

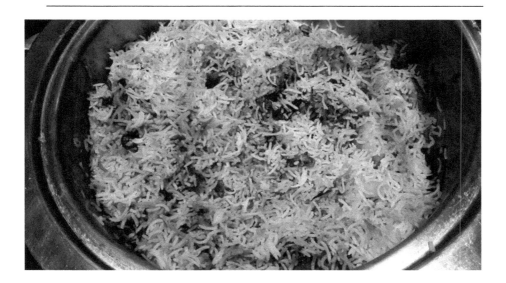

Prep Time: 10 Minutes

Cook Time: 30 Minutes

Total Time: 40 Minutes

Servings: 4

Ingredients

- 1 1/4 pounds chicken breast or lamb, cut into bite-size pieces
- 2 tablespoons olive oil
- 4 pods green cardamom
- 10 whole peppercorns
- 1 cinnamon stick
- 1 bay leaf
- 1-star anise
- 1 pinch saffron (small)
- 1 cup diced onion
- 2 tablespoons fresh grated ginger
- 2 cloves garlic, minced

- 1 cup basmati rice
- 1 1/4 cup stock, chicken or beef
- 1/3 cup sultanas (golden raisins)
- 1/3 cup chopped dried apricot
- 1/2 cup almonds or cashews
- Salt
- Chopped cilantro for garnish

Instructions

- In a large stockpot heat 2 tablespoons of oil over medium heat. Add the cardamom, peppercorns, cinnamon, bay leaf, anise, and saffron. Stir for 2-3 minutes, to allow the spices to release their flavor. Then add the onions.
- Sauté for 2-3 minutes. Add the ginger and garlic and sauté for another 2 minutes. Add the chicken to the pot. Salt liberally and cook for 1-2 minutes.
- Next, add the rice and stir to coat it in oil. Add the stock and bring to a boil. Once boiling pour the sultanas on top, cover, and reduce the heat to low.
- Cover and steam the rice for 15 minutes. Then remove from heat. Stir in the chopped apricots and nuts, then cover again.
- Allow the Yakhni Pulao to sit another 5 minutes, covered. Serve with cilantro sprinkled on top!

Nutrition

- Calories: 572kcal, Carbohydrates: 60g, Protein: 38g, Fat: 20g, Saturated Fat: 2g, Cholesterol: 90mg, Sodium: 465mg, Potassium: 922mg, Fiber: 5g, Sugar: 11g, Vitamin A: 450iu, Vitamin C: 7.3mg, Calcium: 102mg, Iron: 2.4mg

37.   Pesto Chicken Kebabs With Cool Quinoa Pilaf

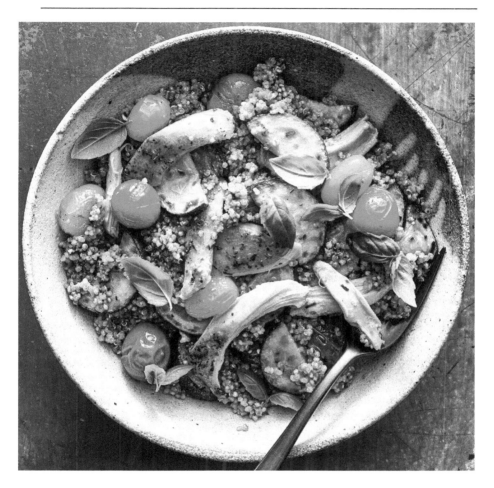

Prep Time: 15 Minutes

Cook Time: 30 Minutes

Total Time: 45 Minutes

Servings: 6

Ingredients

- 1 tablespoon SimpleNature Organic Coconut Oil, or olive oil
- 4 Kirkwood Never Any! Fresh Boneless Skinless Chicken Breasts
- 1/3 cup Priano Genovese Pesto Sauce
- 1 1/2 cups SimplyNature Organic Quinoa
- 1 1/2 cups chopped cucumber
- 1 1/2 cups chopped fresh strawberries
- 1 mango, peeled and chopped
- 3/4 cup Southern Grove Slivered Almonds
- 1/2 cup chopped red onion
- 1/4 cup chopped cilantro
- Salt and pepper, Stonemill Sea Salt Grinder, and Whole Black Pepper Grinder
- 12 wooden skewers

Instructions

- Preheat the grill to medium-low heat, about 300 degrees F. Soak wooden skewers in water for 20+ minutes so they don't burn up on the grill. Cut the chicken breasts into 1-inch cubes. Place them in a bowl and toss the chicken pieces with pesto sauce. Set aside.
- Place the slivered almonds in a medium saucepot and set over medium heat. Toast the almonds for 3-5 minutes, stirring every minute, until they are golden brown. Then pour the almonds onto a plate.
- Set the same saucepot back over medium heat. Add the oil and quinoa. Allow the quinoa to toast for 2-3 minutes. Then add 3 cups of water and 1 teaspoon salt. Cover the pot with a lid and bring to a boil. Simmer the quinoa for 15-20 minutes, until the water has absorbed and vent holes form on the surface of the quinoa. Remove from heat and let the quinoa rest for 10 minutes, covered. Then fluff with a fork and pour the quinoa into a large salad bowl to cool.
- Meanwhile, slide the chicken pieces onto 12 skewers. Grill the chicken kebabs for 5 minutes. Carefully flip them over and grill another 5-7 minutes. Move the kebabs to a platter and cover loosely with foil to keep warm.

- While the kebabs are grilling, add the chopped cucumber, red onion, strawberries, mango, toasted almonds, and cilantro to the cooled quinoa. Toss well. Taste, then salt and pepper as needed.
- Serve the pesto chicken kebabs warm over the cool quinoa pilaf.

Nutrition

Calories: 455kcal, Carbohydrates: 41g, Protein: 27g, Fat: 21g, Saturated Fat: 4g, Cholesterol: 49mg, Sodium: 220mg, Potassium: 809mg, Fiber: 6g, Sugar: 7g, Vitamin A: 665iu, Vitamin C: 34.3mg, Calcium: 110mg, Iron: 3.2mg

38.   Caribbean Chicken Curry Sheet Pan Dinner

Prep Time: 15 Minutes

Cook Time: 30 Minutes

Total Time: 45 Minutes

Servings: 4

Ingredients

- 2 pounds boneless skinless chicken thighs (4-6 pieces)
- 1 red onion
- 1 red bell pepper
- 1 large sweet potato
- 1 tablespoon fresh thyme leaves (or 1 teaspoon dried)
- 1 1/2 teaspoon curry powder
- 1 teaspoon Chinese five-spice powder, or allspice
- 1/4 - 1/2 teaspoon cayenne pepper
- 13 ounces unsweetened coconut milk (1 can)
- 2-3 cloves garlic
- 2 tablespoons fresh grated ginger
- 2 tablespoons honey
- 1 1/2 teaspoons corn starch or arrowroot powder
- Salt and pepper

Instructions

- Preheat the oven to 425 degrees F. Lay a large rimmed 18x13 inch "half sheet" baking pan out and spray with nonstick cooking spray. Place the chicken thighs on the baking sheet.
- Peel the onion, and cut it into quarters. Then slice into 1/4 inch wedges. Seed the bell pepper, and slice into 1/4-inch strips. Then cut the strips in half. Peel the sweet potato, and cut into 1/4-inch rounds. Then cut all the rounds into quarters. Spread the vegetables out on the baking sheet in a single layer.

88

- Sprinkle the top of the chicken and vegetables with curry powder, Chinese five-spice, cayenne, thyme, 1 1/2 teaspoons salt, and black pepper to taste. Bake for 20 minutes.
- Meanwhile, place the coconut milk, peeled garlic cloves, ginger, honey, and cornstarch in the blender. Puree until smooth.
- After 20 minutes, remove the sheet pan from the oven. Pour the coconut mixture over the top of the chicken and veggies. Jiggle the pan a little to help mix the roasted spices into the coconut milk. Then place back in the oven for 10 minutes, or until the curry sauce simmers. Serve warm.

Nutrition

Calories: 288kcal, Carbohydrates: 13g, Protein: 23g, Fat: 15g, Saturated Fat: 10g, Cholesterol: 107mg, Sodium: 118mg, Potassium: 530mg, Fiber: 2g, Sugar: 7g, Vitamin C: 23.4mg, Calcium: 36mg, Iron: 2.3mg

39. Skinny Chicken Enchilada Dip

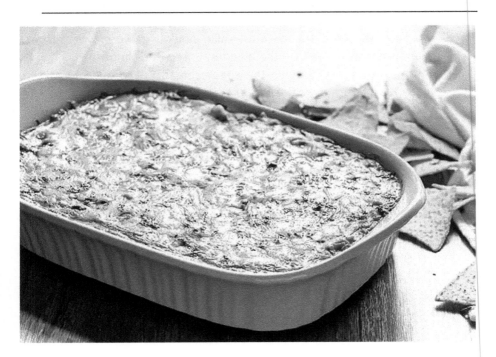

Prep Time: 8 Minutes

Cook Time: 30 Minutes

Total Time: 38 Minutes

Servings: 12

Ingredients

- 16 ounces Old El Paso Traditional Refried Beans (1 can) or fat-free
- 2 cans Old El Paso Red Enchilada Sauce (10-ounce cans) or one 19-ounce can
- 8 ounces light cream cheese
- 1 1/4 cups reduced-fat Mexican-style shredded cheese, separated
- 2 cups chopped cooked chicken
- Scallions or cilantro for garnish
- Baked veggie chips

Instructions

- Preheat the oven to 350 degrees F. Spread the Old El Paso Refried Beans in the bottom of an 8- or 9-inch baking dish. Cover the beans with chopped chicken. Then top the chicken with 1 cup shredded cheese.
- Place the cream cheese in a food processor (or blender.) Puree to soften. Then add in the Old El Paso Red Enchilada Sauce and puree until smooth.
- Pour the creamy enchilada sauce over the shredded cheese. Bake for 30 minutes. Then pull the dip out of the oven and sprinkle the top with the remaining 1/4 cup shredded cheese. Garnish with fresh chopped scallion or cilantro if desired. Serve warm with baked veggie chips or raw vegetables.

Nutrition

Calories: 177kcal, Carbohydrates: 5g, Protein: 9g, Fat: 13g, Saturated Fat: 6g, Cholesterol: 47mg, Sodium: 365mg, Potassium: 73mg, Fiber: 1g, Sugar: 1g, Vitamin C: 0.3mg, Calcium: 118mg, Iron: 0.7mg

40.   Indian Grilled Chicken

Prep Time: 15 Minutes

Cook Time: 40 Minutes

Total Time: 55 Minutes

Servings: 8

Ingredients

- 3 1/2 pounds boneless chicken breast
- 1/4 cup oil
- 1 lemon, zested, and juice from half
- 2 tablespoons Garam Masala
- 2 tablespoons chopped cilantro
- 2 cloves garlic, minced
- 1 tablespoon freshly grated ginger
- 1 teaspoon cumin
- 2 teaspoons salt
- 1/2 teaspoon ground black pepper
- 1/2 teaspoon cayenne pepper

Instructions

- Preheat the grill to medium heat. Place the chicken in a large baking dish.
- In a separate bowl, combine all the remaining ingredients and mix well. Rub the mixture over the chicken, coating completely.
- Grill the chicken for approximately 5-6 minutes per side, turning once. (Grill 35-40 minute total for bone-in chicken.) Serve warm!

Nutrition

Calories: 297kcal, Carbohydrates: 1g, Protein: 42g, Fat: 12g, Saturated Fat: 1g, Cholesterol: 127mg, Sodium: 812mg, Potassium: 738mg, Fiber: 0g, Sugar: 0g, Vitamin A: 120iu, Vitamin C: 3.5mg, Calcium: 14mg, Iron: 0.9mg

41. 295. Vietnamese Cold Chicken Salad (Goi Ga)

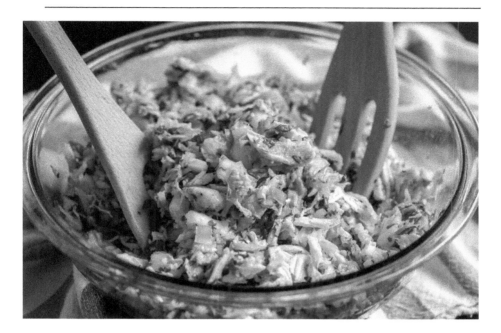

Prep Time: 10 Minutes

Total Time: 10 Minutes

Servings: 8

Ingredients

For The Vietnamese Cold Chicken Salad:

- 6 cups shredded napa cabbage
- 2 1/2 cups cooked shredded chicken, cold (use leftovers or a rotisserie chicken)
- 3/4 cup fresh mint, roughly chopped
- 3/4 cup shredded carrots
- 1/2 red onion, peeled and sliced thin
- 1/2 cup fresh cilantro, roughly chopped

- 1/2 cup chopped roasted peanuts (cashews for paleo-friendly)

For The Nuoc Cham Dressing:

- 1/4 cup fresh lime juice
- 1/4 cup water
- 3 tablespoons honey
- 2 tablespoons fish sauce
- 1 teaspoon chili garlic sauce

Instructions

- Place all the salad ingredients in a large bowl.
- In a small bowl, whisk together the lime juice, water, honey, fish sauce, and chili garlic sauce.
- When ready to serve, pour the dressing over the salad and toss well.

Nutrition

Calories: 167kcal, Carbohydrates: 14g, Protein: 13g, Fat: 7g, Saturated Fat: 1g, Cholesterol: 33mg, Sodium: 202mg, Potassium: 348mg, Fiber: 2g, Sugar: 9g, Vitamin A: 2315iu, Vitamin C: 25.2mg, Calcium: 51mg, Iron: 0.9mg

42.   Chicken Broccoli Quinoa Skillet

Prep Time: 10 Minutes

Cook Time: 25 Minutes

Total Time: 35 Minutes

Servings: 8

Ingredients

- 1 1/2 pounds boneless skinless chicken breast
- 1 1/4 cups dried quinoa
- 3 1/2 - 4 cups chicken broth
- 2 cups small broccoli floret
- 1 bell pepper (yellow or orange), seeded and chopped
- 4 garlic cloves, minced
- 1 cup pecan pieces
- 3/4 cup dried cranberries
- 3/4 cup chopped scallions
- 1 tablespoon olive oil
- 1/2 teaspoon crushed red pepper
- Salt and pepper

Instructions

- Place a large skillet or saute pan over medium-high heat. Once hot, add the oil and chopped bell pepper. Saute for 2 minutes. Then add the broccoli florets. Stir and saute another 3-4 minutes, until the broccoli is partially softened. Remove all veggies from the skillet and set them aside.
- Next add the whole chicken breasts, garlic, quinoa, 3 1/2 cups chicken broth, 1/2 teaspoon salt, 1/2 teaspoon crushed red pepper, 1/4 teaspoon black pepper. Stir and bring to a simmer. Once the quinoa is boiling, lower the heat and simmer until the chicken is cooked through, the broth is evaporated, and the quinoa spirals have separated about 18-20 minutes. Add another 1/2 cup broth if needed.

- Remove the chicken from the skillet. Chop the chicken and add back to the skillet. Then toss in the sautéed vegetables, pecan pieces, cranberries, and scallions. Taste, then salt and pepper as needed. Serve warm!

Nutrition

Calories: 476kcal, Carbohydrates: 42g, Protein: 32g, Fat: 20g, Saturated Fat: 2g, Cholesterol: 72mg, Sodium: 151mg, Potassium: 879mg, Fiber: 6g, Sugar: 12g, Vitamin A: 1030iu, Vitamin C: 56.9mg, Calcium: 62mg, Iron: 3.1mg

43. Southwestern Vegetable & Chicken Soup

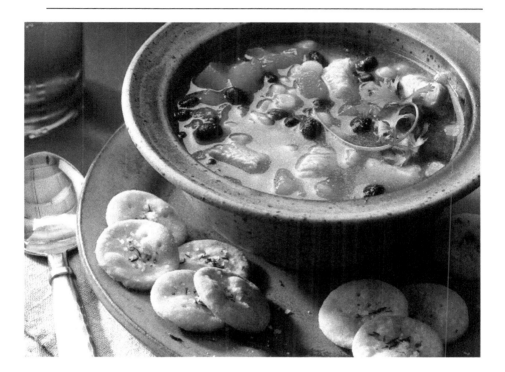

Total: 1 hr 30 mins

Servings: 8

Ingredients

- 2 medium poblano peppers
- 2 teaspoons canola oil
- 12 ounces boneless, skinless chicken thighs, trimmed, cut into bite-size pieces
- 1 1/2 cups chopped onion (1 large)
- 1 1/2 cups chopped red or green bell pepper (1 large)
- 1 ½ cups green beans, cut into 1/4-inch pieces, or frozen, thawed
- 4 cloves garlic, minced

- 1 tablespoon chili powder
- 1 ½ teaspoon ground cumin
- 6 cups reduced-sodium chicken broth
- 1 (15 ounces) can of black beans or pinto beans, rinsed
- 1 (14 ounces) can diced tomatoes
- 4 cups chopped chard or spinach
- 1 ½ cups corn kernels, fresh or frozen
- ½ cup chopped fresh cilantro
- ½ cup fresh lime juice, plus lime wedges for serving

Instructions

- To roast poblanos: Position oven rack about 5 inches from the heat source; preheat broiler. Line the broiler pan with foil. Broil whole poblanos, turning once, until starting to blacken, 8 to 12 minutes. Transfer to a paper bag and let steam to loosen skins, about 10 minutes. When the poblanos are cool enough to handle, peel, seed, stem, and coarsely chop; set aside.
- Meanwhile, heat oil in a large soup pot or Dutch oven over medium-high heat. Add chicken and cook, turning occasionally, until lightly browned, 3 to 5 minutes. Transfer to a plate and set aside.
- Reduce the heat to medium and add onion, bell pepper, green beans, and garlic. Cook, stirring, until beginning to soften, 5 to 7 minutes. Stir in chili powder and cumin and cook, stirring, until fragrant, about 30 seconds. Stir in broth, beans, tomatoes, and the chopped poblanos; bring to a boil. Reduce heat to maintain a simmer and cook, stirring occasionally, until the vegetables are tender, about 15 minutes.
- Add the reserved chicken and juices, chard (or spinach), and corn; return to a simmer and cook for 15 minutes more to heat through and blend flavors.
- Top each portion with 1 tablespoon each cilantro and lime juice; serve with lime wedges.

Nutrition

213 Calories; Protein 16.6g; Carbohydrates 24.9g; Dietary Fiber 5.9g; Sugars 6.7g; Fat 6.4g; Saturated Fat 1.3g; Cholesterol 39mg; Vitamin A Iu 2806.4IU; Vitamin C 72.3mg; Folate 44.5mcg; Calcium 79mg; Iron

2.8mg; Magnesium 72.2mg; Potassium 778.5mg; Sodium 385.5mg; Thiamin 0.5mg.

44. Chicken & Spinach Soup With Fresh Pesto

Total: 30 mins

Servings: 5

Ingredients

- 2 teaspoons plus 1 tablespoon extra-virgin olive oil, divided
- ½ cup carrot or diced red bell pepper
- 1 large boneless, skinless chicken breast (about 8 ounces), cut into quarters
- 1 large clove garlic, minced
- 5 cups reduced-sodium chicken broth
- 1 ½ teaspoons dried marjoram
- 6 ounces baby spinach, coarsely chopped
- 1 15-ounce can cannellini beans or great northern beans, rinsed
- ¼ cup grated Parmesan cheese
- ⅓ cup lightly packed fresh basil leaves
- Freshly ground pepper to taste
- ¾ cup plain or herbed multigrain croutons for garnish (optional)

Instructions

- Heat 2 teaspoons oil in a large saucepan or Dutch oven over medium-high heat. Add carrot (or bell pepper) and chicken; cook, turning the chicken and stirring frequently until the chicken begins to brown, 3 to 4 minutes. Add garlic and cook, stirring, for 1 minute more. Stir in broth and marjoram; bring to a boil over high heat. Reduce the heat and simmer, stirring occasionally, until the chicken is cooked through, about 5 minutes.
- With a slotted spoon, transfer the chicken pieces to a clean cutting board to cool. Add spinach and beans to the pot and bring to a gentle boil. Cook for 5 minutes to blend the flavors.
- Combine the remaining 1 tablespoon oil, Parmesan, and basil in a food processor (a mini processor works well). Process until coarse

paste forms, adding a little water and scraping down the sides as necessary.

- Cut the chicken into bite-size pieces. Stir the chicken and pesto into the pot. Season with pepper. Heat until hot. Garnish with croutons, if desired.

Nutrition

Calories: 227; Protein 19.4g; Carbohydrates 18g; Dietary Fiber 6g; Sugars 1.7g; Fat 9.1g; Saturated Fat 2g; Cholesterol 28.5mg; Vitamin A Iu 3865.7IU; Vitamin C 29.4mg; Folate 76.7mcg; Calcium 92.8mg; Iron 2.1mg; Magnesium 43.7mg; Potassium 524.6mg; Sodium 211.4mg; Thiamin 0.1mg.

45. Lemon Chicken Orzo Soup With Kale

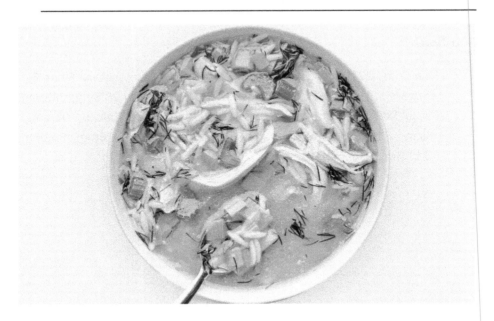

Active: 40 mins

Total: 40 mins

Servings: 6

Ingredient

- 2 tablespoons extra-virgin olive oil, divided
- 1 pound boneless, skinless chicken breasts, trimmed and cut into 1-inch pieces
- 1 teaspoon dried oregano and/or thyme, divided
- 1 ¼ teaspoons salt, divided
- ¾ teaspoon ground pepper, divided
- 2 cups chopped onions
- 1 cup chopped carrots
- 1 cup chopped celery

- 2 cloves garlic, minced
- 1 bay leaf
- 4 cups unsalted chicken broth
- ⅔ cup orzo pasta, preferably whole-wheat
- 4 cups chopped kale
- 1 lemon, zested and juiced

Instructions

- Heat 1 tablespoon oil in a large pot over medium-high heat. Add chicken and sprinkle with 1/2 teaspoon each oregano (and/or thyme), salt, and pepper. Cook, stirring occasionally until lightly browned, 3 to 5 minutes. Using a slotted spoon, transfer the chicken to a plate.
- Add the remaining 1 tablespoon oil, onions, carrots, and celery to the pan. Cook, scraping up any browned bits until the vegetables are soft and lightly browned, 3 to 5 minutes. Add garlic, bay leaf, and the remaining 1/2 teaspoon oregano (and/or thyme). Cook, stirring, until fragrant, 30 to 60 seconds.
- Add broth and bring to a boil over high heat. Add orzo. Reduce heat to maintain a simmer, cover, and cook for 5 minutes. Add kale and the chicken, along with any accumulated juices. Continue cooking until the orzo is tender and the chicken is cooked through, 5 to 8 minutes more.
- Remove from heat. Discard bay leaf. Stir in lemon zest, lemon juice, and the remaining 3/4 teaspoon salt and 1/4 teaspoon pepper.

Nutrition

Calories: 245; Protein 21.1g; Carbohydrates 24.2g; Dietary Fiber 5.4g; Sugars 4.6g; Fat 7g; Saturated Fat 1.2g; Cholesterol 41.8mg; Vitamin A Iu 4723.8IU; Vitamin C 22.2mg; Folate 39.4mcg; Calcium 56.7mg; Iron 1mg; Magnesium 30.8mg; Potassium 480mg; Sodium 638.9mg.

46. Tinola (Filipino Ginger-Garlic Chicken Soup)

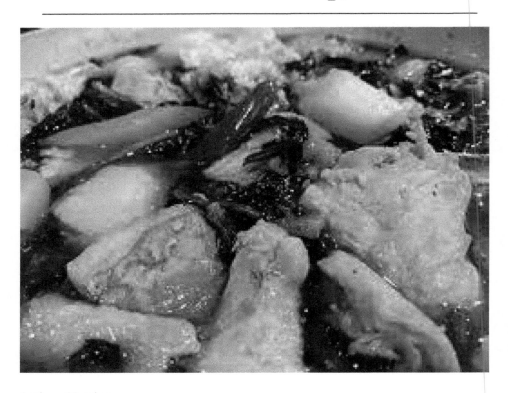

Active: 45 mins

Total: 45 mins

Servings: 4

Ingredients

- 3 tablespoons canola oil or avocado oil
- ½ cup chopped yellow onion
- ¼ cup thinly sliced fresh ginger
- 6 cloves garlic, minced
- 1 pound boneless, skinless chicken thighs, trimmed and cut into 1/2-inch pieces

- 4 cups low-sodium chicken broth
- 1 ½ cups peeled and cubed green papaya or chayote
- 2 cups chopped malunggay leaves or bok choy leaves
- 1 tablespoon fish sauce
- ¼ teaspoon salt
- ¼ teaspoon ground black pepper

Instructions

Heat oil in a large pot over medium heat. Add onion, ginger, and garlic; cook, stirring until the onion starts to turn translucent, about 3 minutes. Add chicken and broth; cook, stirring, until the chicken is just cooked through, about 5 minutes. Add papaya (or chayote), malunggay (or bok choy), fish sauce, salt, and pepper; continue simmering until the vegetables are tender and the flavors have melded, about 5 minutes more.

Nutrition

Calories: 344; Protein 27.4g; Carbohydrates 14.2g; Dietary Fiber 1.9g; Sugars 6.1g; Fat 20.5g; Saturated Fat 3.6g; Cholesterol 75.5mg; Vitamin A Iu 2134.5IU; Vitamin C 52.1mg; Folate 56mcg; Calcium 82.8mg; Iron 2.3mg; Magnesium 51.9mg; Potassium 634.2mg; Sodium 663mg; Thiamin 0.1mg.

Lightning Source UK Ltd.
Milton Keynes UK
UKHW020750030621
384855UK00001B/57